In every uninhibited labour there is a marked restlessness: the woman walks, stands, squats, kneels, lies down, and moves her body freely to find the most comfortable and appropriate positions. There can be no fixed position for a natural healthy labour and birth when a woman follows her own instincts – for birth is active, involving a succession of changing positions, and is not a passive 'confinement'.

This is the first tenet of the Active Birth Movement Manifesto and is the conviction that runs through this practical, compassionate and informative handbook.

Many women are still being denied the right to choose an active birth. Women often experience difficulty and conflict when attempting to give birth in upright, squatting or kneeling positions. *Active Birth* is written to help you prepare for an active childbirth. It will enable you to develop all your resources for dealing with the experience of birth and it aims to bring back commonsense to childbirth, which has often been overlooked in the development of obstetrics.

Janet Balaskas is a counsellor for childbirth, trained with the National Childbirth Trust, and was a founder member of the London Birth Centre and the Active Birth Movement.

D1353317

ACTIVE BIRTH

JANET BALASKAS

London
UNWIN PAPERBACKS
Boston   Sydney

First published by Unwin Paperbacks 1983

UNWIN ® PAPERBACKS
40 Museum Street, London WC1A 1LU, UK

Unwin Paperbacks
Park Lane, Hemel Hempstead, Herts HP2 4TE, UK

George Allen & Unwin Australia Pty Ltd,
8 Napier Street, North Sydney, NSW 2060, Australia

© Janet Balaskas 1983

British Library Cataloguing in Publication Data

Balaskas, Janet
    Active birth.
1. Childbirth
I. Title
618.4   RG651
ISBN 0-04-612033-5

Set in 10 on 11 point Times by V & M Graphics Ltd, Aylesbury, Bucks
and printed in Great Britain
by Guernsey Press Co. Ltd, Guernsey, Channel Islands

Contents

Acknowledgements

We would like to thank all of the mothers and their families who so generously shared their experiences with us, who taught us so much and contributed the labour reports and photographs in this book.

Thanks are also due to Laura McKechnie for the illustrations and Anthea Sieveking for the cover photograph.

For classes in the Balaskas method of preparation for Active Birth contact:

The Active Birth Movement
32 Willow Road
London NW3 (Telephone: 01-794 5227)

Preface

I have never been an athletically inclined person. Given any excuse I prefer not to exert myself. During my first pregnancy I attended preparation classes and was hoping for a natural birth. When Nina was born I was active until strong labour began and then I lay passively in bed, semi-reclining. By concentrating on my breathing and with the help of a dose of muscle relaxant, an episiotomy and enormous effort, I managed to give birth to her spontaneously.

I was introduced to active childbirth during the birth of my second daughter, Kim. Throughout the pregnancy I had been stretching regularly and had benefited enormously from the deep relaxation of tension in my body. When it came to the labour, I again took to my bed, propped up by pillows and focused my attention on my breathing. I made very slow progress dilating, despite my carefully nurtured ability to keep calm and centred.

Our family doctor, fresh from a working holiday in Botswana, where he had watched African women giving birth, came in and advised me to get out of bed and try some squatting.

That got the labour going without any more problems and it dawned on me that it was necessary to open my body and to be in harmony with gravity in order to give birth fully. However, it wasn't easy for me to squat and I resolved there and then to improve my squatting before my next labour.

My husband, Arthur, who taught me to stretch and has a deep understanding of the human body, had been quietly telling me for years that squatting is the logical position for any woman to adopt while giving birth and is the most important position to practise during pregnancy.

Although I was not yet fully convinced, I practised squatting and stretching every day.

During my third labour, I kept active; walking, squatting and kneeling.

I gave birth to my son, Jed, kneeling.

It was a marvellous experience. I had an entirely new sense of control and knew instinctively what to do. I was up within hours of the birth and felt none of the aches and pains I had for a week or two after my previous births, despite the fact that he was almost a 10-lb baby. I was astonished how fit and well I felt after the birth and suffered no exhaustion or depression in the following months.

Throughout these years I had trained with the National Childbirth Trust as a counsellor for childbirth and had also been stretching regularly with all the pregnant women who came to preparation classes in my home. A few of them had some experience of stretching or yoga, but most of them were completely new to this sort of bodywork. The women were of different ages from 19 to 42 and some were in better shape than others. My husband and I were surprised to see how their bodies readily responded to stretching, how their flexibility improved and how their courage, health and happiness increased.

Most of them had uncomplicated, completely natural, joyous births and those that came up against problems and took advantage of obstetric help, usually felt that they had done their best. All recovered in a remarkably short space of time.

After Jed's birth, I began to teach women with a new confidence to prepare for an active birth by stretching and practising the natural birth positions throughout pregnancy. We also spent hours discussing different aspects of birth, labour and motherhood, often together with their husbands.

The experiences of these women have added to my personal conviction and won support from their midwives, doctors and obstetricians.

Many women enjoy the benefits of stretching so much that they are back in the mother and baby stretching sessions two to three weeks after birth. This is so, not only in the case of the mother who has a normal, problem-free birth but also for those who have needed the help of forceps or Caesarean section.

Over the years I have seen that active labour and the adoption of a natural, upright or crouching birth position is the safest, most enjoyable, most economical and sensible way for the majority of women to give birth. There is no disruption of the normal physiology of labour, no interference with the hormonal balance, post-natal depression is rare and problems with breastfeeding and mothering are less likely.

The majority of labours – managed well – should be uncomplicated. No special equipment is needed and the birth can take place in the simplest environment or in the most sophisticated hospital delivery room.

Active birth is natural and instinctive. Left to her own devices, it is the way a woman will spontaneously behave during labour. In preparing a woman for an active birth my aim is to help her get in touch with her own birth-giving instinct.

Giving birth is essentially a natural bodily function, which occurs quite spontaneously and involuntarily at the end of pregnancy. It is part of a continuous evolution which begins with love-making and conception and ends in the gradual growth of independence of the child from his mother during the first few years of life.

The whole process of conceiving a baby, being pregnant, giving birth and mothering is part of the sexual and spiritual life of a woman and is basically rooted in the natural and undisturbed unfolding of a series of physiological events.

The best way in which a woman, entering into motherhood, can prepare herself is from her own body.

The stretching exercises we recommend are not unnatural movements imposed upon the body. On the contrary, they are instinctive and simple movements we could all make with ease. It is a kind of physical 'remembering' rather than a system of exercise. In fact many of the exercises in this book came from our observations of the movements made by our children when they were very young. By watching them we realised how stiff we have become, how we have lost contact with the range of movement nature intended us to have.

A toddler will squat with ease for a long time, feet flat on the ground, back straight and rising up from this position when he learns to walk.

It is well known that the more civilised we become the more we forget our natural habits. Today we are able to ensure a reliable medical back-up for all women in the event of complications and the mortality rate has been improved by the life-saving techniques of modern obstetrics. However, I have seen, all too often, in my practice, how the widespread use of routine obstetric technology, inappropriately applied to normal labour, disturbs the natural birth process and causes many of the problems it was designed to prevent. In some hospitals birth has become an abdominal or vaginal extraction conducted on a conveyor belt.

The result is that most women are completely out of touch with their own instinctive ability to give birth and midwives are losing their intuitive skills as they depend more on technology.

Many women have never seen a birth or even held a baby by the time they enter motherhood. The natural skills of giving birth and mothering are no longer handed down from woman to woman, generation to generation.

We can regain a link with our primitive female heritage by re-educating our bodies in the habits, movements and postures which are instinctive to the child-bearing woman.

In pregnancy the whole tendency of the body is towards health and growth and it is a unique opportunity for a woman to work on herself.

The main concern of this book is with normal birth and the common variations from the norm which can usually be dealt with, without obstetric intervention.

Women who have prepared in this way and then found themselves faced with an unexpected complication, or have needed the help of pain-relieving drugs, often find ways of successfully combining active birth with obstetric procedures.

I hope that this book will help to bring to light the simple common sense of childbirth which has somehow been obscured in the advance of modern obstetrics and will help women to rediscover their own inner resources for giving birth to their babies.

Foreword

Here is a new and important voice in childbirth. Janet Balaskas is speaking to those women who want to grow in self-awareness and to use their bodies actively in labour. In her childbirth classes Janet Balaskas stands for activity rather than passivity, for movement rather than immobilisation and a woman's right to choose whatever position she finds comfortable throughout labour and delivery.

The teaching in this book is revolutionary. Yet it is age-old. All over the world and throughout recorded history women have chosen upright positions to give birth and it is only we in the West who have had the extraordinary notion that a woman should lie on her back with her legs in the air to deliver a baby.

But to get women upright is to do much more than help them find a comfortable posture. It is to turn them from passive patients into active birth-givers. It is to challenge the whole obstetric view of birth in Western society. This is based on the assumption that childbirth is a medical event which should be conducted in an intensive care setting. The whole of pregnancy is seen as a pathological condition terminated only by delivery. The modern high-tech obstetrician actively manages labour with all the technology of ultrasound, continuous electronic monitoring and oxytocin intravenous drip. Many obstetricians have never had the opportunity to see a truly natural birth. To turn the process of bringing new life into the world into one in which a woman becomes simply the body on the delivery table rather than an active birth-giver is a degradation of the mother's role in childbirth.

We are now beginning to discover the sometimes long-term destructive effects on the relationship between a mother and her baby and on the family of treating women as if they were merely containers to be relieved of their contents and of concentrating attention on a bag of muscle and a birth canal, instead of relating to and caring for the person of whom the uterus and the vagina are a part.

'Bonding' is a fashionable term today. In many hospitals special time is devoted for bonding and there must be few midwives and obstetricians who would not claim that they consider bonding important. But everything that happens after delivery is the outcome of what has gone before. Bonding is either spontaneous and easy, or made virtually impossible by the atmosphere at delivery and by the care a woman is given as a *person*, not merely a 'para 1', an elderly primigravida, a maternal pelvis, a contracting uterus or a dilating cervix.

The way we give birth is important to all of us because it has a great deal to do with the kind of society we want to live in, the significance of the coming to birth of a new person and a new family.

When we hand over responsibility for choosing between alternatives on the basis of what we believe to be right, we hand over responsibility for the quality of the society we, and our children, must live in.

Sheila Kitzinger

1
What Is An Active Birth?

If you give birth actively you will stand, walk, sit, kneel, squat and assume any upright position you choose in the early part, or first stage of labour. As you approach the expulsive or second stage of labour, up to and including the actual birth of your child, you will use natural expulsive positions, like squatting, sitting, or kneeling either upright or on your hands and knees (usually supported).

An active birth involves you giving birth through your own will and determination, having the complete freedom to use your body as you choose, and to find any method of supporting yourself. It is an attitude of mind as well as an attitude or position of body, and is not merely a vaginal extraction or a passive delivery.

You may be like some women who, left to themselves, will instinctively know what to do; but then again you may be like most women who, having no example to follow, need to be made aware of the possibilities of using various upright and crouching positions.

You will find practising these birth positions and movements appropriate to pregnancy and will learn best how to relax and make yourself comfortable. You will be cultivating the natural and right body habits for pregnancy and birth. Birth is essentially a biological and not a technological function. The comfort and well being of you and your child are of prime importance. An active birth is more comfortable, safer and more efficient than its opposite – a passive birth. This is supported by the many scientific studies comparing women who are active in labour with those in the passive, recumbent position.

The Question of Birth Positions

A growing number of women, midwives, nurses, obstetricians and prenatal teachers are questioning positions that characterise labour and birth and the passive, patient-orientated role demanded of women in contemporary maternity care. The specific practice that is being criticised is the almost exclusive use of lying down (recumbent) positions for childbirth known as supine, dorsal or lithotomy positions. Whereas there is more than sufficient evidence that upright birth positions, i.e. kneeling, sitting, standing, and squatting are more advantageous to both mother and child.

Position and movement in labour is an area of fundamental importance which has been almost completely neglected by birth attendants in the management of labour, and therefore prenatal teachers in the preparation of women for birth. The choice of position determines the training of obstetricians, midwives and nurses. It also determines the approach of the staff and the kind of space needed in maternity care settings for women in labour.

Modern Western Practice

Obstetric practice in the Western world is normally regarded as a medical if not a surgical procedure. The normal practice in most hospitals is to place you, when you are in labour, in bed on your back; at best propped up by pillows into a semi-reclining position. Just before the time of actual birth you are transferred to a delivery room and placed on an obstetric table where monitors, drips, and anaesthetic can be applied and where forceps delivery, vacuum extractor (venteuse) and episiotomy can be performed conveniently and conventionally. The teaching hospitals' approach to training in maternity care determines the choice of your birth position. The teaching and its pupils predetermine that you lie down.

There is no doubt that the most direct influence in promoting and demanding the recumbent position for labour and delivery is the specific training of physicians, midwives and nurses in obstetric practices such as:

● labour and delivery seen as an illness in which the attendants and their attendant technology are in control rather than you yourself, your instincts and your biological body
● the use of sedatives, analgesics and anaesthesia during labour and delivery
● the need to assess foetal heart tones, uterine and other vital signs during labour
● the use of forceps and/or episiotomy for delivery.

No one will deny the enormous advantages of the safety net of modern obstetrics when problems occur which may threaten the life of you or your baby, or both. However, the vast majority of labours are uncomplicated and it is clear that common sense in the management of labour has been completely obscured by the routine application of interventive obstetrics to normal labour, resulting in a great increase in the number of forcep deliveries and Caesarian sections (recent statistics in Ottawa, Canada, reveal that the majority of babies are delivered by forceps, and in the USA the Caesarian rate is almost 30 per cent). The rigid insistence of making women in labour lie on their backs may contribute much to these figures.

Historical Evidence

Historical studies show the prevalent use of vertical positions – kneeling, squatting, standing or sitting postures – with many variations and as many methods of support.

There is evidence going back thousands of years of the bodily positions taken in childbirth. The head of a silver pin from Luristan in Iran, first millennium BC, depicts a squatting mother. The remains of a clay statue of 5750 BC from a shrine at Çatal Hüyük, a Copper Age (chalcolithic) city in Turkey, shows a goddess giving birth in the same position, as does an 8½-inch Aztec fertility stone figure from Mexico. A relic of the Mound Builders of eastern Arkansas, a pre-Columbian culture of unknown date, shows a woman squatting with her hands on her thighs. The Egyptian hieroglyph meaning 'to give birth' shows a mother squatting.

A relief from the temple of Kom Ombo, a town on the Nile in Upper Egypt, shows a woman giving birth in the kneeling position. Birth in the same position can be seen in a marble figure from Sparta, about 500 BC. In ancient China and Japan women customarily gave birth in the kneeling position on a straw mat. All scenes, of course, depict only the final birth, but positions used during the rest of labour can also be traced.

In the Old Testament, Exodus, chapter I, verse 16, states:

When ye do the office of a midwife to the Hebrew women, and see them upon the stools ...

A Corinthian vase depicts a woman in labour seated on a birthchair.

An early Greek relief and a Roman marble base-relief both show a woman giving birth on a stool supported by two assistants.

The birthstool was recommended for uncomplicated labours by Soranus in the early second century AD and by many subsequent writers. It was described as 'In a form like a barber's chair but with a crescent-shaped opening in the seat, through which the child may fall.' The first birthstools must have been rocks or logs of wood, developing over time into complex, adjustable chairs with many varied devices.

From the Birthchair to Bed and Delivery Table

In the Western world the birthstool or chair remained indispensably part of the equipment of most midwives up to the middle of the eighteenth century. Each wealthy household had its own stool, while among the poor a stool was transported from house to house. The birthstools of royalty were carved and ornamented with jewels. Dutch, German and French sixteenth-century drawings show the great use of birthstools, as do Chinese drawings of the same period. Even today a birthchair is still used by some Egyptian women.

The first record of a woman lying down for birth is of Madame de Montespan, mistress of Louis XIV, who lay down in a recumbent position so that he could watch the birth from behind a curtain. In the mid-seventeenth century in France two brothers named Chamberlain invented the forceps. The best position for forceps delivery is to have the woman lying down. This invention was jealously guarded by the Chamberlains who performed their deliveries shrouded by black drapes. This firmly entrenched the obstetric fashion for ladies of quality to give birth in recumbent positions and the obstetrician took over from the midwife in the birth chamber. In the same century François Mauriceau became the leading figure in French obstetrics. He scorned the use of the birthchair and advocated childbirth in bed lying on the back. As forceps gained popularity the birthchair lost favour and by the end of the eighteenth century little more was heard of it.

In the nineteenth century Queen Victoria was the first woman in England to use chloroform while giving birth. Delivery under anaesthetic further installed the lying down position on the back or on the side. Birth positions which lend themselves more easily to the convenience of the attendants who perform these procedures became the only choice and the practice of confining a woman to bed for the major part of her labour and then on to an obstetric table for delivery eventually spread throughout the Western world.

The birthchair had given way to the bed and the delivery tables of the nineteenth and twentieth centuries. Women were now flat on their backs, a position that made them passive and controllable, and that offered a fine view to the attendant but was in total defiance of the active forces of gravity and the joyous independence that comes from naturally and instinctively giving birth actively on one's own two feet.

Ethnological Evidence

Primitive tribes have adopted various birth positions through the customs of their tribe, but more important, by their instinct. Some forty positions have been recorded, and their relative merits have been much disputed. Women of different tribes squat, kneel, stand, incline, sit or lie on the belly, so, too, do they vary their positions in various stages of labour and in difficult labours.

Dr G. J. Englemann, in his book *Labour Among Primitive Peoples*, written in 1883, was one of the first to investigate the various positions assumed in labour or childbirth by early people, and he found that the four principal positions were squatting, kneeling (including the all-fours and knee-chest positions), standing and semi-recumbent.

Ethnologists entirely confirm the evidence of the historians. Whatever the race or the tribe under observation, African, American, Asian and so on, the same upright positions always predominate – standing, kneeling, sitting and squatting with a great variety of means of support. Figures reveal that throughout the world today, for the most part, women still labour and deliver in some form of upright or crouching position, usually supported.

Recent Studies

Documented evidence has been available for over fifty years as to the physiological advantages of labour in upright, crouching positions. Certain principles of physics apply to childbirth which are denied or negated when a woman gives birth lying down. The facilitating influence of squatting positions has also been radiographically confirmed in the 1930s. It was shown that the cross-sectional surface area of the birth canal may increase by as much as 30 per cent when a woman changes from lying down on her back to the squatting position. And it is some twenty years since Scott and Kerr demonstrated the disadvantages of having the weight of a pregnant uterus pressing down on the back. Lying supine the weight of the contracting uterus reduces the placental blood flow by compressing the large artery of the heart (the descending aorta) and the large veins leading to the heart (inferior vena cava). This is a hard clinical fact which should not be ignored by anyone involved with childbirth.

Most recent studies have revealed definite advantages to a woman when walking about and assuming upright positions during labour. The few, and they are a very small minority, who have not found any measurable advantage, all conclude that there is definitely no disadvantage to being active and using upright positions during labour.

The majority of studies have established a control and an experimental group. This has usually required that the control group remain supine or in some recumbent position in bed and that the experimental group assume an upright position, sitting, squatting, kneeling or walking about. Other studies which seem more convincing have used women as their own controls by asking them to alternate every thirty minutes between two positions – horizontal and upright – during the first and second stages of labour. These alternative means of examining the effect of position during labour both reveal similar positive results in favour of active upright labour and deliveries.

In the last ten years many studies have been carried out in various parts of the world.

In 1977 a study in Birmingham Maternity Hospital compared a group of women who walked about during labour with a group that lay down horizontally throughout most of labour.

The results showed that the duration of labour was significantly shorter, the need for analgesics far less, and the incidence of foetal heart abnormalities markedly smaller in the ambulant group than in the recumbent group.

Women walking about also experienced less pain with uterine contractions and felt more comfortable upright.

They concluded convincingly that walking about during labour, especially early labour, should be encouraged.

In Latin America Dr Roberto Caldeyro-Barcia organised a

collaborative study involving two maternity hospitals. Vertical labour positions (sitting and standing) and horizontal positions (side lying and lying on the back) were studied. Their effects on the labour and on the condition of the baby were compared.

In 1972 in America Dr Isaac N. Mitie of Indiana compared women in the second stage half of whom were lying down and the other half in sitting positions.

Dr Yuen Chou Lui headed a study of sixty women in labour in two hospitals, one in New York city and the other in Washington.

These are a few of the many recent studies giving positive evidence of the benefits of walking about and using upright labour and birth positions. Most studies confirmed that uterine contractions were stronger and more efficient in dilating the cervix.

Results of Modern Research

Most studies reported that when upright and moving about the following advantages ensued:

1 The intensity (strength) of uterine contractions was found to be greater.
2 Greater regularity and frequency of uterine contractions.
3 The dilation or opening of the cervix (the neck of the uterus) was greater.
4 More complete relaxation between contractions.
5 The pressure of the resting phase between uterine contractions was consistently higher.
6 The first and second stages of labour were shorter (some comparative studies showed over 40 per cent shorter time in the upright group).
7 Greater comfort, less stress and pain and so decreased requirement for analgesics.
8 Improved condition of the newborn.
9 Women felt they were contributing something to their labour and felt relieved from the boredom of lying down connected to equipment.

Why is Active Birth Better?

What explains the fact that women have easier labours when they move about and assume upright crouching positions? These recent studies suggested that in the upright positions:

1   The pull of gravity, i.e. the earth's gravitational force, assists uterine contractions and bearing-down efforts by adding pressure. It is easier for any object to fall towards the earth's surface than to slide parallel to it (Newton's law of gravity), so that it is mechanically more advantageous to expel an unborn baby towards the earth than to expel it along the horizon.

2   The drive angle of the uterus, i.e. the angle between the long axis of the unborn baby's spinal column and that of the mother's spinal column, is less when upright so demanding less effort for the uterus.

3   The increased pressure of the abdominal wall and the diaphragm on the uterus increases the resting phase pressure upon the uterus.

4   The entrance of the baby's head or presenting part to the inlet of the mother's pelvis is easier and the head's direct application to the mother's cervix is assisted, because the pelvic inlet points forward and the outlet faces downward producing a convenient angle for descent. With each contraction of the uterus the unborn baby has a tendency to sink and this sinking is towards the mother's cervix.

5   There is an improved placental circulation giving a better oxygen supply to the foetus.

Disadvantages of Lying Down in Labour

Dr Peter Dunn, Consultant Senior Lecturer in Child Health at Southmead Hospital in Bristol, wrote in *The Lancet* in 1976 of the recumbent position for labour, 'No animal species adopts such a disadvantageous posture during such an important and critical event.'

Lying on one's back is the one position that causes compression of the major abdominal blood vessels along the spinal column. Compression of the large artery of the heart (descending aorta) can cause foetal distress by hindering blood circulation around the uterus and the placenta. Compression of the large veins leading to the heart (inferior vena cava) blocks the returning blood flow, contributing to hypertension and maternal haemorrhage.

Lying on one's back does not take advantage of the mobility of the pelvic bones and the suppleness of the pelvic muscles. It ignores the help of flexing the knees and hips, i.e. the acute angle made by bringing the knees towards the chest, which opens and alters the shape of the pelvis.

When lying flat on the back without any trunk flexion, the direction of the uterus's force conflicts with the direction of descent of the head or any other presenting part. This wastes energy and effort and increases the duration of labour.

When lying down for delivery the perineum stretches unevenly at the expense of the posterior part, often demanding an episiotomy and certainly increasing stress and pain.

Implications

Based on research findings, various up-to-date studies and ancestral instinct, it is foreseeable that certain changes with respect to labour and birth positions are inevitable in the management of labour and in the preparation of women for childbirth.

As changes in positions help to increase the strength and effectiveness of contractions, allowing a woman to be up and to walk about in early labour, especially if there are no complications, seems rational and good practice. A woman's own instincts dictate to her that she should move around. Standing, walking about, and assuming various sitting, kneeling and squatting positions, with any suitable means of support, causes the uterus to exert more pressure on the foetus and in turn on the cervix. Women should be guided more by their own feelings, comfort and need rather than by hospital convenience and obstetric fashion. Freedom of one's body is necessary to find those positions which traditionally have been used to facilitate labour and delivery; positions which will assist one to attain maximum comfort, relaxation, ease and control.

There is an infinite range of possible positions and no constant chronological order. It is the need to search for the most effective, efficient and comfortable positions that is common. The common need amongst women instinctively to keep changing positions will one day have to be universally recognised. This involves a different attitude to the management of labour, to maternal care generally and to antenatal preparation.

A prospective mother needs not only knowledge of pregnancy, labour and delivery, the growth and development of babies, but also adequate physical preparation concerning the effects of varying upright positions and the cultivation of ease and comfort in them, so that she can actively and effectively help herself during labour.

Squatting

Change of position is more important than a single optimal or best position during labour. It is unlikely that any woman would elect to remain in one position throughout labour. However, squatting is closest to nature's laws and is known as the physiological position.

A birth position is physiologically effective:

when there is no compression on the vena cava,
when the pelvis becomes fully mobilised.

Supported squatting seems to be especially efficient at the end of delivery. The squatting position produces:

1 Maximum pressure inside the pelvis.
2 Minimal muscular effort.
3 Optimal relaxation of the perineum.
4 Optimal foetal oxygenation.

A supported squat may be essential in a breech delivery as it reduces delay between delivery of the umbilicus and the head.

Another useful position is the all-fours position. The presenting part rotates inside the pelvis more easily when a woman is on all-fours.

None of the women in all the recent studies were prenatally prepared to gain ease and comfort in squatting, kneeling, crouching and all-four positions. How much better would the upright groups of women have fared if they had had the additional physical preparation. (A controlled study of this kind has not yet been done.)

Ideal Maternity in Pithiviers, France

Michel Odent and his staff provide a setting for women to be active in labour at his maternity unit at Pithiviers in France. For over fifteen years in his unit women in labour have had the freedom to follow their instincts in walking about and finding positions that are suitable and comfortable. He and his midwives together with expectant mothers have discovered many means of physical support during labour and delivery which have proved over the years to be a tremendous advantage in easing labour and especially delivery. They do not use foetal monitoring, pethidene, epidurals or forceps. Few episiotomies are given and induction is very rare. Their concept of obstetrics, i.e. non-disturbance is very different from conventional practice aimed at control. Also the material and the human environment is very different.

In this unit there are about 1,000 deliveries a year. Professional care is the responsibility of Dr Odent and six midwives. The midwives work in pairs forty-eight hours at a time followed by four days off.

Each woman is given her own room throughout her stay and there are few rules. As labour advances she walks to the birth room, which has a low-level platform and a wooden squatting stool with many cushions. There she is allowed to remain active and change her position as many times as she wishes.

Most women prefer to walk about, sit on the birthstool, kneel on all-fours, squat and lean on their husbands or the midwives for physical support. Water is regarded as important and women, if they like, may take a warm bath or relax in a small plastic swimming pool which is available. No drugs are used. The membranes are not artificially ruptured. Most women adopt an upright position for delivery usually a supported squat, others give birth on the birthstool or on the low double bed and some give birth in water. With the appropriate supported squat and the gentle control of crowning there are no unnecessary perineal tears and episiotomies are rare.

After the birth, the baby's bath and the delivery of the placenta, the mother walks with her husband, and her newborn back to her own room. Of the 1,000 births that took place there in 1981 only eight newborns needed intensive care.

Here is a maternity-care setting close to ideal. It has the safety of hospital delivery as well as the relaxed atmosphere of a comfortable and homely birth room. It is free of frustrating regulations, the normal labour ward rush and most important a sick-role attitude towards a woman in labour. They have a positive approach to an active, natural outcome. The attendants are well known to the mother and give her constant attention during labour and delivery.

Fathers participate and give their support. Women are given the freedom to move and adopt any position they find comfortable and the minimum use of drugs and interventions during labour are needed.

If the majority of women at Pithiviers can experience active birth safely and naturally in such a unit why not elsewhere?

Results of 898 births at Pithiviers in 1980

		per thousand
* Perinatal deaths	8	10
Caesareans	44	5.0%
Episiotomies	71	8.0
Vacuum extractions	57	6.3
Manual removal of placenta	10	1.1
Total previous Caesareans	26	2.9
Vaginal deliveries after previous Caesareans	18	2.0
** Transfers to pediatric unit	15	1.7
Forceps	0	

* All deaths after 6 months gestation.
** Severe jaundice, malformations and premature.

Your Responsibility

If the freedom to move about and adopt upright positions makes sense to you and you want to give birth actively but do not have a maternity unit like that run by Michel Odent, how can you go about it? Obviously you will have to make the possibility of an active birth your own responsibility. You will have to prepare your body to cultivate ease and comfort in upright birth positions as well as find (whether you wish to give birth at home or in hospital) a doctor or obstetrician and midwife who will support you in giving birth actively without the conventional intervention.

In parts of Britain, Europe, North and South America, Australia, New Zealand and elsewhere small numbers of women, doctors, midwives and antenatal teachers are teaching and putting active birth into practice. Unlike Pithiviers where an enlightened obstetrician and his midwives initiate the active birth movements, these small groups springing up everywhere spread their message by word of mouth.

These women have the proof of experiencing an active birth without drugs, without episiotomies and without tears. They prepare themselves to give birth actively by finding antenatal teachers who encourage them in this and they find doctors and midwives, maternity units and staff who are prepared and willing to allow them to move about and use upright positions. If you want to give birth actively you will have somehow to make contact with one of these groups who help themselves to give birth actively and naturally. If this is not possible you will have to convince your doctor or midwife or whoever to allow you to follow these suggestions.

Suggestions for Labour

During the first stage while the cervix is dilating it is usually best to be upright and walking about.

During the second stage, standing or kneeling with the upper body leaning well forward during contractions helps to complete rotation of the head.

At the end of the second stage, supported squatting seems to be the most effective and comfortable during contractions.

Squatting, especially supported, gives the greatest increase of pressure in the pelvic cavity with a minimal muscular effort and optimal relaxation.

2
Stretching for Pregnancy

Stretching is a system of exercises which will help you to rediscover the natural range of movement your body is designed to make. In our modern technological society there is a hidden epidemic of stiffness, caused partly by the stresses and strains of life and partly by poor physical education and the comforts of modern living. We are so out of touch with the full range of movement we are capable of making that our muscles and joints have become tense and stiff. Stiff muscles lose their elasticity. They 'shrink' and the movement of the joints they work becomes restricted and restricting. We end up carrying a load of unnecessary tension around with us, actually bound up in our musculature.

Try this
Stand upright with your feet one foot apart and your knees straight. Bend forwards towards the floor, moving from your hips and keeping your back straight. Hold for a few seconds and then come up.

You will feel a stretching sensation in the muscles at the back of your legs as the movement causes them to lengthen and relax. You are probably wondering why this is painful, if the muscles are relaxing. The reason is that it is so long since you have made the full movement that the hamstring muscles at the back of your legs have shortened and lost their elasticity, restricting your ability to move forward. Nature has designed your body to be able to fold over like a jackknife, with your stomach and chest flat against your thighs, and the palms of your hands flat on the ground in front of you.

You will probably find that this state of chronic tension exists throughout your body to some degree. This stiffness, of which we are usually quite unaware, hampers our capacity to turn inwards and enjoy deep states of consciousness and lessens our ability to use and enjoy our physical potentials.

The most effective way to become more relaxed and supple is by beginning to make the neglected movements we were designed by nature to make. It is simply a matter of spending some time each day practising them. Gradually stiff muscles will lengthen and tension will relax.

The result will be a healthy, enjoyable and energetic pregnancy and the rediscovery of a new and unique intimacy with your own body, which you were always intended to have. The stretching exercises are a system of movements designed to relax and lengthen all the muscles of the body in a safe, passive and non-strenuous way which harnesses the help of the forces of gravity and your natural potential for movement. Pregnancy is a time when one is particularly receptive to change and growth and there is a natural inclination towards health. A variety of hormones help to soften your joints and make them more supple. Relaxation is something you can cultivate in these months, it is a unique and marvellous time to work on yourself – to turn inwards.

'I'd never exercised before and found some of the positions quite hard to start with, but gradually, with practice, I loosened up. I concentrated mainly on about 6 or 7 exercises which I tried to do every day.'

The Benefits of Stretching in Pregnancy

- As your muscles become more elastic and your joints more supple, the balance of the muscle-pulls that support and move your body improves. Muscles work in teams – while one team is relaxing and lengthening the other is contracting and shortening. By balancing the opposing teams of muscle-pull, your joints articulate better and your posture automatically improves. This ensures that you are carrying your baby correctly and will help to prevent backache.

- During pregnancy the weight you are carrying puts extra strain on your lower back. As well as poor posture, backache is often caused by poor tone in the buttock muscles which support the back. Stretching exercises help to strengthen these muscles and often backache can improve or disappear quite dramatically after a few weeks of exercising.

  'I found that the most comfortable ways to rest, watch T.V. or read were either to sit in the butterfly position on the floor or on all fours leaning on cushions. The latter position was invaluable whenever I got backache.'

- As you become familiar with the exercises you will find movements which alleviate the minor discomforts of pregnancy, such as heartburn, pain in the hip joints or in the ribs or cramps in the legs.

- Your circulation depends upon your muscles. Blood vessels run through your muscles acting as pumps and return blood from your lower body back up to your heart. If a muscle is stiff then the blood vessels running through it are constricted and your blood circulation (and indeed indirectly the circulation to your baby in the womb) will be restricted. By stretching regularly you can help to ensure that your baby is getting everything he needs to grow healthy and strong. Problems associated with poor circulation – varicose veins, haemorrhoids (piles) or fluid retention – will be prevented or improved. Stretching also tends to lower the blood pressure and can often help to prevent problems associated with rising blood pressure. (See chapter 9.)

- Stretching helps to combat fatigue. If muscles are stiff and movement is restricted the flow of energy is 'blocked'. After a session of exercise you will feel invigorated and refreshed, more energetic and alive. Over time this will increase and your pregnancy can be a time when you feel healthier and more energetic than ever.

- The most comfortable positions in pregnancy will naturally extend into the labour itself. So without needing to think about it very much you will have cultivated ease and comfort in the natural positions for birth used by women through the ages. You will be able to move freely and instinctively like a primitive woman – your body will know what to do. Stretching during pregnancy will help you to be more deeply in touch with your own body and with your essentially primitive consciousness. It will be easier to behave involuntarily and to surrender to the powerful forces within your body during labour.

   'When the contractions became very strong I knelt upon the delivery bed and leant over a very large firm cushion – this seemed to be a natural position for me to adopt, as I had used it so much in late pregnancy.'

   'Stretching prepared me to relax as much as possible during and between contractions, to stay squatting, and to give birth in a position which allowed me to be in control.'

- As stiffness lessens during the hours spent in stretching, you will be helping your body to become free of pain. You will learn how to become familiar with the discomforts and even the pain of going beyond your usual limits. As labour and birth demand a going beyond one's normal limits, positioning your body to do this physically during pregnancy prepares you gradually for this, so that when labour arrives you are familiar with this kind of effort. Stretching teaches you to surrender to the forces within your body. This is the best possible practice for labour, and will help you to cope with the intensity of the sensations of your contracting uterus.

'By exercising I learned how to be at one physically and emotionally with the changes which would inevitably lead to the birth of my child. The teaching enabled me to "go with" my body, even when the pain was a burden. I was physically and also theoretically prepared for everything that was to happen to me and I approached the final events with excitement and real confidence.'

● Whatever happens during labour and delivery, even if complications arise, regular stretching throughout pregnancy is the best way to prepare for a speedy recovery and return to normal.

Basic Anatomy

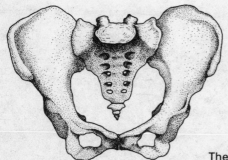

The female pelvis

Your pelvis is the part of your body most directly involved with giving birth. It is the bony passage through which your baby will pass as it is born. During pregnancy your body produces several hormones which soften the joints in order to increase their flexibility and assist the birth of your child. By stretching you can make the most of this natural flexibility and be at your physical best for giving birth.

Try this

a. Kneel on the floor and explore your pelvis from the outside.

Place your hands on your hips and find the illiac crests – two bony points at your sides – and follow their curved rim with your thumbs round to the back. Feel your pubic bone in front, your sacrum and coccyx at the back.

b. Sit on your hands and feel your two buttock bones.

c. Kneel, then lift up one foot so that you are half kneeling and half squatting. Explore your pubic arch. Feel its curve extending from your buttock bones under your pubic bone. Your baby's head will pass under this arch as it is born.

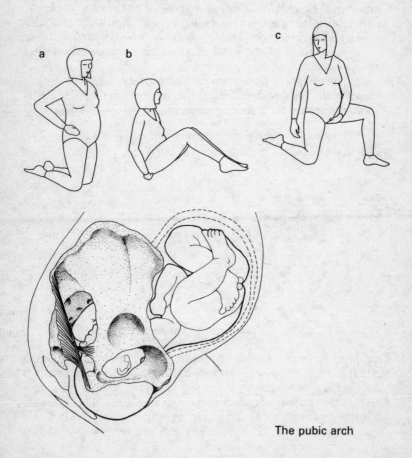

The pubic arch

Your pelvis is shaped internally like a curved funnel, exactly the right shape to accommodate your baby's head as it passes through during labour. From above you can see the pelvic inlet in which your baby's head will engage ready to be born; and from underneath the outlet through which it passes at birth.

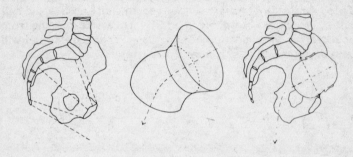

The pelvic canal

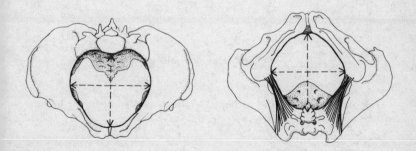

Pelvic inlet and outlet

Your pelvis has 4 major joints.

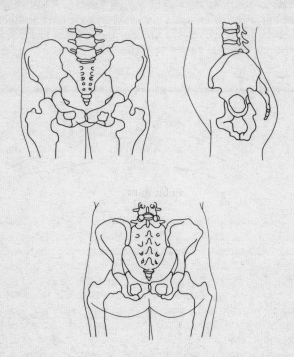

Pelvic bones and joints

The pubic joint in front can open as much as ½ inch during labour to make room for your baby's head.

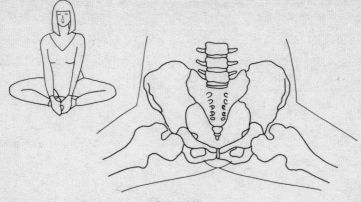

Pubic joint

The two sacro-illiac joints are at the back. These joints expand from side to side and also move in a pivot-like way to increase the area of the pelvic canal and assist the passage of your baby.

When you bend forward, as in squatting or kneeling, your sacrum and coccyx lift up and this opens and expands the pelvic outlet. When you bend backwards or recline, this has the effect of closing the pelvic outlet and narrowing the space by as much as 30 per cent. This is one of the reasons why reclining is the worst position to adopt for giving birth.

'When I was in labour I went for a bath at one point. There I made a big discovery for myself – I sat on my sacrum in the normal way and I could feel it closing up – I lay back into the water and there was a contrast between the lovely feeling of the water and the discomfort of the position – so of course I turned over and knelt in the bath. I was very interested to actually feel *the closing of my pelvis.'*

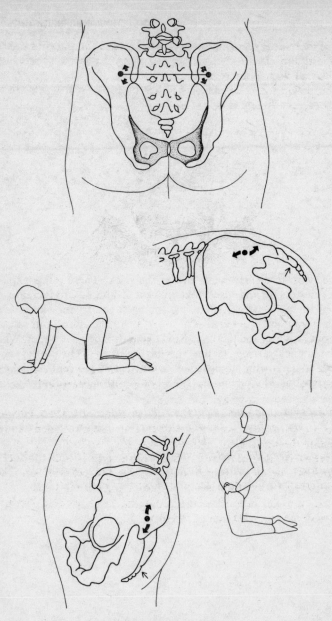

The sacro-illiac joints

The sacro-coccygeal joint is between your coccyx and your sacrum. This joint loosens during pregnancy so that your coccyx moves out of the way as your baby is born.

The pelvic joints are held together by ligaments which are like strips of very strong elastic.~

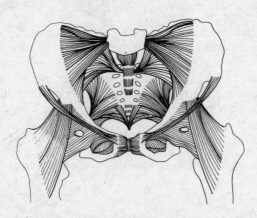

The pelvic ligaments

The sources of power of this part of your body are the muscles which are attached to the bones and bring about movement at the joints when they contract and relax.

The pelvic muscles include the buttock muscles at the back which provide strength and support for your spine and upper body and are especially important during pregnancy.

At the base of your pelvis, attached to the area around the outlet is a sling-like band of muscles which form the pelvic floor. These surround and form the base of the anus, vagina and urethra.

These muscles support all the abdominal contents and your baby will pass through them as he is born.

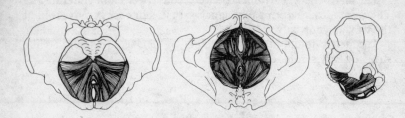

The pelvic floor

The uterus is a powerful muscle shaped like a hollow bag within which your baby is growing. It is attached by strong ligaments to the pelvic bones.

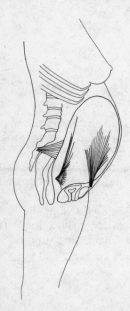

The uterus

Other muscles which are attached to your pelvis are the abdominal muscles, back muscles and the leg muscles.

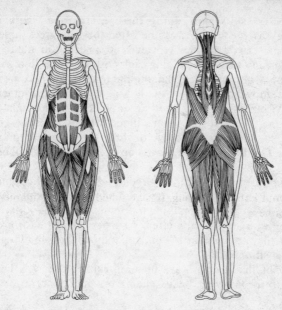

Muscles which attach to the pelvis

Your pelvis supports and distributes the weight of your upper body and protects and supports your uterus and growing baby.

Correct flexion of the pelvis during pregnancy is crucial for good posture, for the safe carriage of your child and will help to ensure a good birth.

The stretches for pregnancy concentrate on the pelvis and include all the major joints of the body.

Introduction to Stretching

Choose a time of day when you have an hour to yourself – first thing in the morning or perhaps the last thing at night. It is best not to eat a large meal beforehand.

For best results start doing these exercises as early in your pregnancy as possible. Any time after the 12th week unless your doctor advises you sooner. However, it is never too late to benefit. Start off in any easy way holding each position for as long as you are comfortable, gradually lengthening the time as you become familiar with the movements. Start with a few of the movements and gradually build up until you are able to go through the full programme. The first thing you will feel when you start is your own stiffness, so expect to spend two or three weeks getting to know the exercises. Gradually as you loosen up the movements will become a pleasure.

You will probably find that some of the stretches fit comfortably into your daily habits, that there are some you can practise while watching TV, reading, or talking to friends, and some you would like to concentrate on. All the exercises are perfectly safe for pregnancy and once they are familiar to you, you may safely spend long periods in each position.

If any of the stretches are uncomfortable, after you have tried them out for a while, leave them out and concentrate on the others.

At first you will find that following the instructions carefully, you can go up to a certain point and then you begin to feel the stretch. In each position reach this point and stay with it, breathing deeply, until the stretching sensation eases. Gradually your range of movement will increase and your body will become more flexible and relaxed.

'The exercises I had done during pregnancy were invaluable and made such a difference to the birth and after. I felt more confident and in control of my body and as I write now afterwards I realise what a benefit they have been in getting back to shape afterwards.'

A word of warning

Anyone can benefit from stretching, whether you have exercised before or not, however, if you have a chronic back problem or any complications in your pregnancy, such as a history of miscarriage or cervical stitch, then do check with your doctor first.

Practising these exercises will help to relieve cramps in the calves, backache, varicose veins, haemorrhoids, high blood pressure, sleeplessness, tiredness, nausea and other common complaints of pregnancy, but do read the instructions and the notes on 'caution' before you start each exercise.

Some women find that they are uncomfortable lying on their backs during pregnancy – particularly in the last month. This is because the weight of the heavy uterus presses on the large blood vessels in your abdomen, which slows down your circulation and can cause dizziness. If this happens to you at any stage then roll over onto your side, come up onto your hands and knees (all fours) and in future leave out any exercise which involves lying on your back. However, for most of us this is no problem and lying on the back is very relaxing.

Useful tips

- It is most important for the well being of you and your baby that you attend regular antenatal check-ups with your midwife, doctor, clinic or hospital as well as doing these exercises.

- During your pregnancy try to wear flat-heeled shoes and also use a low stool for squatting on (or a pile of books), or sit on the floor cross-legged instead of on a chair whenever possible.

- It is a good idea to get together with another friend who is pregnant – or perhaps a small group – and practise stretching together. The 'work-out' includes stretches for two. They are equally good for men in case your husband wishes to join you.

- It can be very pleasant to follow your stretching session with a warm bath or shower, or perhaps a swim.

The Stretching Exercises

1 Deep Breathing

Warm up with some exercises for the head and neck. Sit comfortably cross-legged with back straight. Close your eyes, drop your shoulders and allow all tension to melt from your face.

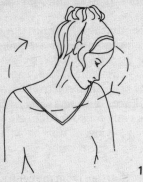

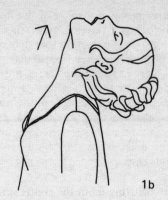

1a

1b

a.   Keeping your body still, slowly begin to rotate your head, breathing comfortably, allowing its weight to carry your neck round the full range of movement to the front then the side, then back to the other side and round again. Do three circles in each direction. And make sure your shoulders are as low as possible.

b.   Starting from the centre, allow your head to drop backwards keeping your mouth wide open. Hold for a few seconds and then, keeping your head back, bring your teeth together so that you stretch the muscles in the front of your neck. Hold for a few seconds and come up slowly.

c.   Drop your head forward. Clasp your hands together and place them behind your head, gently bringing your chin down towards your breastbone. Hold for a few seconds dropping your shoulders and breathing deeply. This relaxes the back of your neck and upper back muscles. Come up slowly. If you have a headache try doing this for 5 or 10 minutes.

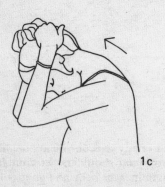

1c

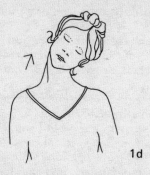 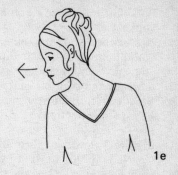

d. Starting from the centre and keeping your body still, lean your head over towards your left shoulder – feel the stretch down the right side of your neck. Come up slowly and then repeat to the right.

e. Starting from the centre, look right round over your left shoulder and then repeat to the right.

How you benefit This routine loosens the joints of your head and neck and lengthens and relaxes the muscles of this area. Regular practice will have a relaxing and calming effect.

Breathing Awareness

You may find it helpful at first to ask someone to read this aloud while you try it. Sit comfortably on the floor. If you prefer, kneel with a cushion between your buttocks and your feet or else simply sit cross-legged. Lean with your back against a wall for support if you like.

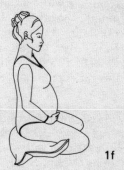

● Close your eyes and try to let go of any tension you are holding. Keeping your back straight, drop your shoulders, let your face become soft, let go of any tension in your belly and your pelvic floor. Sit quietly and become still. Breathe in and out through your nose.

- Now witness your breathing. Don't try to do anything, just centre your attention on the rhythm of your breathing. Notice whether you are breathing with your chest or your belly. Watch the inbreath and then the outbreath.

- Breathe in through your nose, breathe out through your mouth. Pay special attention to the outbreath and breathe out fully, really empty your lungs. Pause for a second or two until you feel the urge to breathe in, then allow your lungs to fill up with air. Continue in this way until you feel really comfortable, allowing your breathing to become slower and deeper, and pausing for a few seconds between breaths.

- Place your hands on your lower belly.
This time, when you exhale, open your mouth and make the sound 'aaaah' coming from as deep and low down as you can. Feel your belly draw inwards as you breathe out and expand as if it were filling up when you breathe in. Always concentrate on breathing out and allow the inbreath to come of its own accord. Repeat several times.

- Now place your hands in your lap or palms-up on your knees, drop your shoulders, sit up straight and make the sound 'mmmm ...' as if humming. Concentrate on the exhalation and pause between breaths. Repeat several times.

- Continue without humming – breathe out slowly through your mouth, breathe in through your nose. Concentrate on the exhalation and pause between each breath.

- Now return to your normal breathing in and out through the nose. Be aware of a still space between each breath. Continue like this for several minutes or longer.

Try to keep your chest still and breathe deeply into your belly. It may take you a few weeks to master this deep breathing – even if you force it a little at first it will soon become second nature. This is not a special breathing technique, it is simply the natural and most deeply relaxing way to breathe.

Many of us, caught up in the hurly-burly of daily life, have forgotten how to breathe like a baby and we breathe too fast, too shallowly and retain one-third of the stale air in our lungs by inhaling too quickly before we have completed the exhalation.

Practise this breathing for a few minutes before you stretch and then breathe deeply through the stretches and you will find that you can breathe through your tension. This is the best possible practice for breathing through the pain of contractions during labour.

'*To breathe deeply was invaluable for control of pain during contractions. The psychological preparation was also very important for me. Practising helped me to believe that I could cope with the pain. This belief gave me confidence and although the pain was excruciating at times, I felt I could get through it.*'

2 The Butterfly

Sit up straight, bringing the soles of your feet together as close to your body as possible. Put your hands behind you, palms down, close to your buttocks to help keep your back straight or else clasp your feet with your hands. If you find this difficult at first, start with your feet 12 inches away from your body and gradually bring them closer.

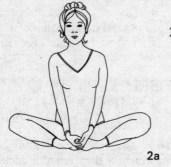

2a

2a. Make small butterfly move-ments with your legs to loosen your hip joints.
After loosening up for a few minutes, you can increase the stretch by working with a partner.

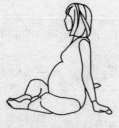

2a RIGHT

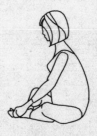

2a WRONG

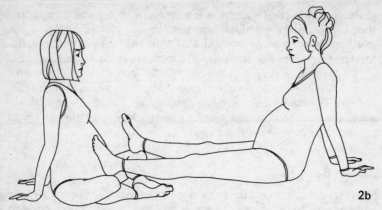

2b

2b. Sit in the position with your back straight and the weight of your trunk supported by your hands. Your partner should sit opposite you, keeping her legs straight, supporting her weight with her hands, and place her feet on your knees.

Hold for a minute or so and then change over.

How you feel   In this position you should feel the stretch mainly in the groin and hip joints and you may also feel it in your knees and ankles.

How you benefit   This stretch is derived from Hatha Yoga and is known to be the woman's position. It is said that if a woman masters this position completely, she is less likely to have any gynaecological problems.

This stretch opens your pelvis from side to side, increasing the flexibility of the pubic and hip joints, widening the front of the pelvic inlet. It also helps to ensure the correct tilt and position of the pelvis.

This exercise also relaxes and tones up your buttock muscles, pelvic floor and uterus and improves the circulation of blood to these areas.

This is a very comfortable sitting position.

The more time you spend in it, the better!

Caution
Make sure your back is straight, lift up from your sacrum and allow your pelvis to tilt forward rather than slump back.

3   Japanese sitting position

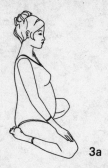

3a

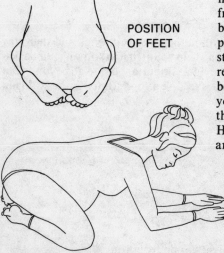

3b

3a. Kneel on the floor with your knees as wide apart as possible, your ankles turned out and your toes pointing towards each other. If you can, sit between your feet, if not, simply sit on your heels.

3b. Open your chest bringing your shoulder blades downwards towards each other. Be aware of your spinal column and imagine a straight line running from your coccyx to the back of your head. With this awareness move slowly forward from the hips, keeping your buttocks down as much as possible and your elbows straight, until your hands reach the floor and you begin to feel the stretch in your groin. If you feel it, stay there and breathe deeply. Hold for a minute or longer and then come up.

POSITION OF FEET

3c

3c.   If you feel no stretch, go down further onto your elbows.

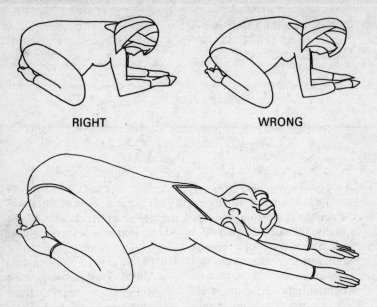

RIGHT   WRONG

3d.   If you still feel no stretch, you may lie flat.

Caution
Go only as far as you can without bending your back and then stay there and breathe into it. It may help you at first to know if your back is straight if you look in a mirror. It is important not to go beyond your limit in this exercise. The idea is to have a good stretch in the groin not to get down low.

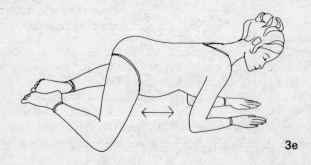

3e

3e. Come forward onto your elbows, lifting your buttocks, open your knees a little further and make a rocking movement backwards and forwards.

This stretch, which we call the frog, was taught to us by our children who all do it quite naturally and often sleep in this position.

How you feel You should be feeling the stretch mainly in the groin and possibly in your knees and ankles. This position encourages a feeling of openness and is good practice for labour.

How you benefit This exercise, practised regularly, will help to restore the full range of movement in your hip joints and groin. It will encourage good posture and open the pelvic outlet. It also allows your belly to hang down and lengthens and relaxes your back, buttock and pelvic floor muscles. This exercise is very helpful in preventing or relieving backache. If your lower back aches or if you get pain from pressure on the sciatic nerve (a sharp shooting pain in the hip – very common in pregnancy) then concentrate on this stretch.

'Although it was difficult at first, I found the Japanese sitting and leaning forward the most comfortable position in late pregnancy. After 2 months my back-ache completely disappeared.'

4 Legs apart on the wall

Caution
During pregnancy, particularly in the last weeks, a few women find that they feel dizzy lying on their backs. This is caused by the weight of the heavy uterus pressing on the large blood vessels in the abdomen and slowing down the circulation. It has been found in practice that, in this position, women who normally cannot lie flat on their backs are often not affected in the same way, as the upright position of the legs alleviates the pressure and improves blood circulation.

To be on the safe side, if you do not feel comfortable in this position after you have tried it once or twice or in late pregnancy, then leave it out and do stretch no. 5 instead. If, however, you are able to do it, this stretch is one of the most relaxing and beneficial, once you get to know it.

'I began Yoga exercises in my fourth month of pregnancy and after a month or two of practising discovered that certain positions were refreshing to do, especially lying with legs apart against the wall.'

Sit down sideways next to the wall so that your hip is touching the wall. Swing round until your upper body is lying flat on the ground and your buttocks are close to or touching the wall.

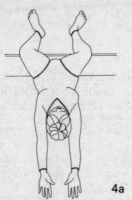

4a

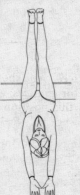

4b

4a. Bend your knees, as if squatting, and lift your arms up over your head. This is the resting position for this stretch.

4b. Straighten your legs and hold for a few seconds until you are used to this position.

4c. Allow your legs to drop open as far as they can, keeping your knees tight and extending your heels, bringing your toes in towards your body. If you can clasp your hands and reverse them. Lift your arms up over your head. Hold for a minute or so, breathing deeply. At first you may only be able to hold this stretch for a few seconds, but when you are used to it you may remain in it for 5–10 minutes. If you need a rest simply bend your knees.

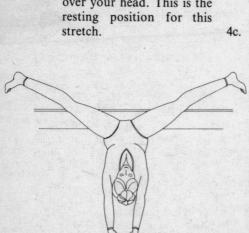

4c

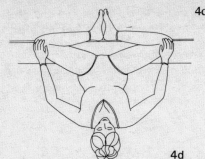

4d. Bring the soles of your feet together close to your body and press your knees towards the wall with your hands. To come out of this stretch, roll over slowly onto your side, wait for a second and then come up on your hands and knees.

4d

How you feel You should feel this stretch in the powerful inner thigh or adductor muscles which run from inside your knees to your pelvis. In this position these muscles are actually lengthening and relaxing. They may feel very painful at first. When these muscles are fully relaxed you can open your legs to almost 180 degrees. In medieval German these muscles were called the guardians of the vagina. Wilhelm Reich called them the morality muscles, as they are the first muscles to tense up against full sexual feeling.

How you benefit In this stretch your spine is completely supported. There is no strain on your abdomen and gravity assists your legs to open. If you practise this for 5 minutes a day, you will soon notice an improvement and it will become less painful. Try massaging these muscles with your hands while in this position. During the course of a pregnancy your legs can drop 6–12 inches, make a mark on the wall where your heels are when you start and observe your improvement!

This stretch, once you get used to it, is extremely invigorating. If you feel tired or exhausted, 10 minutes in this position will work wonders.

This exercise improves the circulation to your legs as the major blood vessels to the legs pass through these muscles. If you suffer from varicose veins or piles, you should practise this stretch at least twice daily. It is one of the few ways to improve varicose veins.

As these muscles relax, your awareness of this part of your body will increase. You will feel more open and you may even feel your enjoyment of the sensations of sex will grow. You will find it easier to cope with and allow the painful, as well as the orgasmic sensations of giving birth.

'*I did not require any analgesia throughout labour. The exercises loosened up my stiff muscles and joints allowing for greater ease during the delivery.*'

'*I was really glad I had prepared my body and loosened it up with all those stretching exercises which had seemed such agony when I first started them.*'

5   Sitting with legs apart

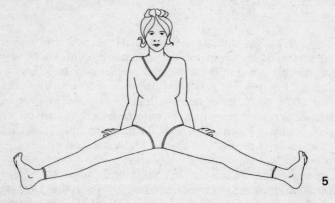

5

Sit on the floor with legs as wide apart as possible. Place the corner of a firm cushion underneath your buttocks and then slide off it, opening your legs to their widest as you do so. Tighten your knees and extend your heels, bring your toes in towards your body. Your back should be straight and you may support yourself by leaning back slightly onto your hands. If you are stretching with a partner, try doing this exercise facing each other and take turns to use your feet to help each other to open further by gently putting a little pressure on the ankles.

How you feel   You should feel the stretch in the inner thigh muscles and in the back of the upper leg.

How you benefit   This stretch is similar to the last one and lengthens and relaxes the thigh muscles. It encourages a feeling of openness and is easy to do while sitting with friends, playing with children or reading.

It is beneficial during pregnancy to sit on the floor rather than on a chair, whenever you can. Many of the stretches, such as this one, make very good sitting positions.

6 Sitting between the feet, leaning back

Caution
Follow the instructions very carefully while learning this stretch. It is important not to go beyond your limit. If your lower back begins to ache this indicates that you are going too far.

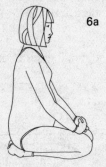

6a

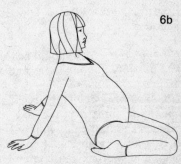

6b

6a. Sit on your heels or between them if you can, with toes pointing towards each other, ankles turned out, and knees together. This is a natural sitting position and you should cultivate ease in it. It stretches your ankles and knees.

6b. Tighten your buttock muscles, then lean back onto your hands, until you begin to feel the stretch in your thighs. Now stop. If you are feeling the stretch, go no further.

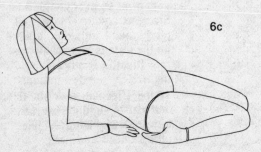

6c

6c. If you are not feeling anything go back onto your elbows, keeping buttocks tight and knees together.

6d

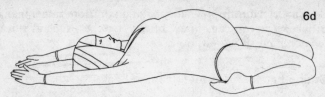

6d. (For the very supple only.) If you still feel no stretch, tighten your buttocks, keep your knees together, lift up your pubic bone and lie down flat.

Hold the position for a few seconds at first and then for 2 or 3 minutes.

How you feel   You should be feeling the stretch in your thighs only, and possibly in your knees and ankles.

How you benefit   This stretch relaxes the front thigh muscles and opens the front of your body, which feels very pleasant. It also extends and lubricates your ankle and knee joints and improves the circulation to your legs. Regular practice will strengthen your lower back and buttock muscles and relax your stomach and digestive system. If you suffer from haemorrhoids (piles) this exercise will help.

This is a good stretch to do after eating and may help to alleviate heartburn or a full feeling.

7   Shoulder Stretch

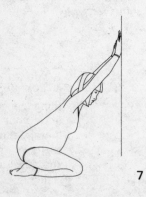

7

- Kneel with knees wide apart, about 1 ft away from the wall, and toes pointing towards each other.
- Drop your shoulders and lift your arms up over your head. Straighten your elbows and place your hands 6 in. apart on the wall as high up as you can. Breathe deeply and hold the stretch for a few minutes.

To be effective your shoulder blades should be gently lowered away from the back of your head and neck.

How you feel   You feel the stretch in the shoulders and upper arms. (Not in your back – if your back aches come closer to the wall.)

How you benefit   This stretch relaxes the shoulders, opens the chest and stretches the muscles which support your breasts.

This is very helpful for stiff shoulders, breathing problems, heartburn or pressure in the ribs, and relieves tension in the upper back.

8   Forward Bend

Stand with your feet slightly apart. They should be pointing straight rather than turned out.

Be aware of your spine – a straight line from your tailbone to the top of your head. Drop your shoulders, bringing your shoulder blades down and together at the back. Open your chest and clasp your hands behind you.

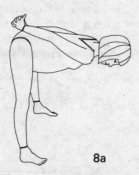 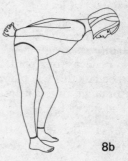

8a

8b

8a. Keeping your back straight, bend forward from the hips until you begin to feel the stretch at the back of your legs. Make your body like an 'L', then simply hang, with back straight, breathing deeply for a few minutes or bounce gently.

8b. Try bending one knee and bouncing gently, alternating knees.

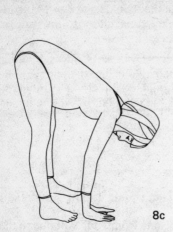

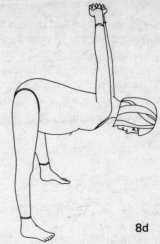

8c

8d

8c. If you can do so without bending your back, place your palms on the floor and hold for a few minutes.

8d. You can also clasp your hands behind your back, keeping elbows straight, and lift them up and back as you bend forward until you feel a stretch in the shoulders. Hold for a minute or so and then come up slowly.

Caution

Take care in your enthusiasm not to go beyond your limit and overbend as this will place strain on your lower back.

You might find it helpful to look in a mirror to check that your back is straight.

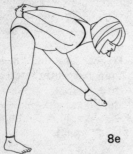

8e. Variation: try doing this exercise with your feet about 3 feet apart and toes turned in. Grip the floor with your toes for balance.

8e

How you feel You will feel the stretch in the hamstring muscles at the back of your legs (a and b) and also in the shoulders (c).

How you benefit   This stretch lengthens and relaxes the hamstring muscles at the back of the legs and improves the circulation to your lower body.

It helps to correct the flexion of the pelvis and is therefore excellent for posture.

Practised regularly this exercise gives you energy and helps to prevent unnecessary fatigue caused by stiffness in the legs.

The last part loosens and relaxes the shoulders and upper back muscles.

9   Standing Stretches

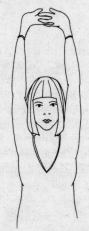

9a

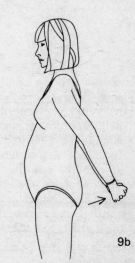

9b

9a. Stand with feet 2 ft apart. Clasp your hands in front of your body, reverse them. Drop your shoulders and then lift up your arms over your head as you inhale and look up to your hands. Keep breathing and hold, then bring your arms down slowly as you exhale. Repeat several times. Feel the stretch in your abdominal muscles and shoulders.

9b. Clasp your hands behind your back, drop your shoulders and then lift up your arms until your shoulder blades meet. Hold for a minute or so, and then let go. This stretch relaxes the shoulders and the muscles which support your breasts.

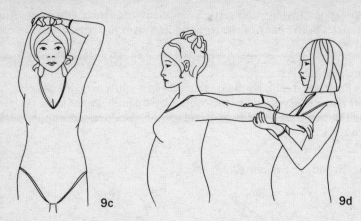

9c.

9d.

9c. Lift one arm up over your head. Bend your elbow so that your hand comes down to the back of your neck. Use your other hand to pull your elbow behind your head to increase the stretch. Hold for a minute or so and then repeat on the other side. This stretch relaxes the shoulders and the rib cage, and helps to relieve pressure in the ribs.

9d. Work with a partner. Stand with feet 2 ft apart. Open out your arms to 180 degrees and keep them at shoulder height. Drop your shoulders. Your partner should then stand behind you and bring your arms towards each other keeping them at shoulder height. Allow your chest to open and breathe deeply. Hold for a minute or so and then let go.

How you benefit This series of stretches relaxes tension in the shoulders and improves the circulation of blood in your chest, head and arms and therefore to your whole body. It opens your chest increasing your lung capacity and improves the circulation of air both for you and your baby. These exercises open the front of the body, making more room and will help to relieve the discomfort of feeling uncomfortably full, heartburn or pains in the ribs which are all common complaints of pregnancy. These stretches also tone up the breasts and the muscles which support them.

Many of us tense up in the shoulders very easily and doing these stretches regularly in pregnancy will help you to feel calm and relaxed now as well as during labour.

10 Calf Stretch

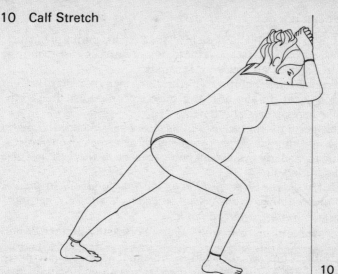

10

Stand facing the wall with your front foot about 1 ft away from the wall and your feet 3 ft apart. Look down at your feet, they should be facing straight ahead.

Lean your upper body forward onto the wall. Rest your head on your arms, keeping neck and shoulders relaxed. Bend your front knee and let your back leg take all your weight. Tighten the knee of your back leg and press your heel into the ground. Hold for a few minutes breathing into the stretch and then change legs. Do this several times.

How you feel You should feel the stretch in the calf muscles of the back leg.

How you benefit You can thank Sebastian Coe, the famous runner, for this stretch which lengthens and relaxes your calf muscles. As these muscles govern the movement of your ankles, this exercise will help to improve your squatting. Try alternating this stretch with squatting and you will find it much easier. This stretch improves the circulation to your legs and feet and is useful particularly during pregnancy when the extra weight you are carrying can put pressure on the blood vessels which supply your legs. Regular practice will prevent cramps in the legs and swollen feet.

Last but not least, this stretch helps to keep your calves shapely.

11 Squatting

Squatting is the most important of all the stretches during pregnancy. It is a natural way to rest and is the first position a baby uses before he or she straightens up and begins to walk.

With the Western habit of using furniture, many of us have lost our ability to squat. In any primitive society people squat frequently, often for long periods at a time.

In this position your pelvis is at its most open and it is the logical position to adopt in order to give birth or to open your bowels. Squatting regularly while you are pregnant is the best possible practice for labour.

'I tried to squat with my feet flat on the floor for about 10 minutes most days and towards the end of pregnancy I could do this pretty comfortably whilst reading a book.'

Caution
If you suffer from varicose veins in the legs or haemorrhoids (piles), or if you have a stitch in your cervix, you should only do easy squatting, either the dictionary squat or use a low stool.

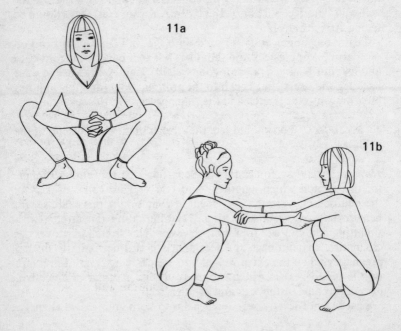

11a

11b

11a. Stand with your feet 2–3 ft apart. Look down at your feet and make sure that they are straight rather than turned out. Keeping your back straight and feet flat, squat down. Clasp your hands, spread your knees apart with your elbows. Squat for a few minutes or as long as you like, if you are comfortable.

11b. If you have already lost your balance you probably have stiff ankles and will find it easier to squat holding onto a friend for support. When you are stretching alone find a strong piece of furniture, door handles or a radiator, you can hold onto for balance. Most people find it necessary to hold on to start with. The exercise is just as beneficial done in this way. It is preferable to hold on rather than to strain.

11c

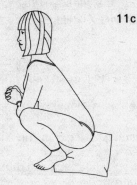

11d

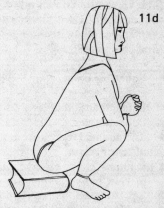

11e

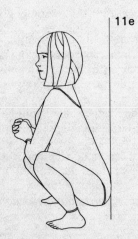

11c. Try placing a firm cushion under your heels.

11d. Place a few large books under your buttocks for support. We call this the dictionary squat and you are meant to remove the books one by one as your squatting improves.

11e. Try squatting against a wall – with just a touch of support on your lower back from the wall.

Try to do the full squatting exercise for at least 5 minutes every day. Instead of sitting on a chair or lounging on the couch try to find a comfortable squatting position using a stool or a pile of books for support, if you need to, so that you can squat for long periods.

During labour you will squat as comfortably as possible using a stool or supported by other people.

'I found squatting the most difficult, though by the end of the 4½ months I found I could squat fairly easily.'

'When I was pregnant I squatted on a hard cushion and because I had used the cushion for practising my breathing and for squatting I went to it in labour without thinking.'

How you feel   You should feel the stretch mainly in the groin but you may also feel it in your ankles, calves and knees.

How you benefit

- Squatting opens your pelvis. The pelvic inlet, canal and outlet are at their widest.
- It lengthens, relaxes and tones your back, buttock and pelvic floor muscles.
- The perineal tissues are at their most relaxed, lessening the chance of tearing.
- It improves the blood circulation to the whole area and thus also to your baby and ensures correct posture.
- Squatting also correctly positions your growing baby and uterus and is very helpful during labour.
- Regular practice of squatting will eradicate constipation and makes one feel very open and in the right frame of body and mind for birth. It is good practice to imagine giving birth while actually squatting. Imagine your uterus opening and your baby's head passing through your pelvis.
- Squatting regularly will encourage the engagement of your baby's head in the pelvic brim (inlet) in the last weeks of pregnancy and will help to prevent complications.
- Even if you don't use this position when you give birth, it is the best possible practice and will ensure a quick recovery.

'My uterus apparently "shrank back in record time" according to the nurses and "check-out lady".'

12 Pelvic Floor Exercises

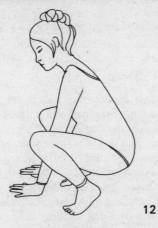

12

12a. With your feet 2 ft apart squat down – this time easy squatting on your toes. Lean forward onto your hands keeping arms and back straight and knees wide apart.

12b. Draw up and tighten your pelvic floor muscles. (The muscles you would normally tighten if you were trying to stop urinating in midstream.) Hold for a few seconds and then slowly release. Repeat several times.

12c. Now try to co-ordinate your breathing with the exercise. Breathe in when you tighten, hold for a second or two and then breathe out slowly as you let go. Imagine that you can feel your baby's head descending in the second stage of labour and 'breathe' your baby out as you release your pelvic floor.

How you benefit   Unlike your uterus, which functions involuntarily, you are able to hold or release your pelvic floor at will. Regular practice of this exercise helps to ensure that you will automatically 'let go' of your pelvic floor muscles each time you breathe out as your baby descends. This lessens the likelihood of a perineal tear.

Your perineum is the fleshy part between your vagina and anus and has an amazing capacity to stretch and fan out as your baby is being born.

This exercise improves the circulation of blood to the area. Tightening and releasing these muscles works rather like rinsing out a sponge in fresh water – each time the muscles release, a fresh supply of blood fills the tissues.

Daily practice will ensure good muscle tone and a speedy recovery after the birth.

13   Positions for Labour

These are a series of movements which are used instinctively by women in labour and are intended as a guide. During labour you will spontaneously discover the sort of movements which make you most comfortable and are invariably best for your baby too. Practise these movements occasionally so that by the time you are in labour they will be second nature. Moving in this way will help you to cope with the pain of contractions and also helps to encourage the dilation of the cervix and the rotation and descent of your baby.

There are infinite variations to these basic movements – you will discover your own way of doing them when the time comes. Try to co-ordinate the movements with deep breathing and imagine that you are breathing through a contraction in labour.

'Kurt put on some quiet music and I felt such a relief and freedom at being able to move about as I felt able to, and be upright and forward or on all fours.'

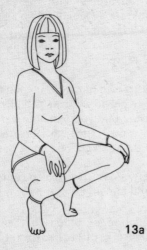

13a.   Squatting
Squat down on your toes and then stand up. Repeat several times. Now try squatting then kneeling and then coming back to squatting. This position is very useful in labour and is a natural position for giving birth.

13a

13b. Standing

Stand with feet apart and rotate your hips in slow sensuous circles rather like a belly dancer. Change to the other direction. Walk up and down and try leaning forward onto a wall, or your partner while making these movements. In the standing position gravity helps your baby to descend and the labour to progress.

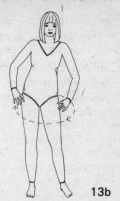

13b

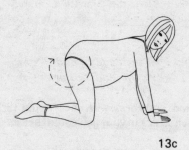

13c

13c. All Fours

Kneel forward on the floor on your hands and knees with knees 1 ft apart. Rotate your hips, making slow, sensuous, circular movements using your whole body while breathing deeply. After a while do the same in the opposite direction. This movement is very useful if your baby is in the posterior position or if your contractions are very intense. It can be used as a position for delivery.

13d. Kneeling

Kneel upright with your back straight and knees slightly apart. Place your hands on your hips and make circular movements like a belly dancer alternating directions.

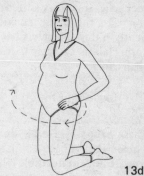

13d

13e. Half kneeling, half squatting

Lift up one knee into the half-kneeling, half-squatting position and rock backwards and forwards. Change feet and repeat on the other side. This movement encourages dilation of the cervix in labour.

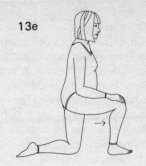

13e

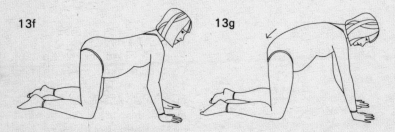

13f   13g

13f and g. Pelvic rocking

Kneel down on the floor on your hands and knees, with knees about 12 in. apart. Tighten your buttock muscles, tuck in your pelvis and then let go. Repeat several times.

During pregnancy your lower back is under considerable strain from the extra weight you are carrying. Tightening your buttock muscles strengthens your lower back and will help or prevent backache. If you are suffering from lower back pain, make a point of practising this often. Tucking in your pelvis ensures correct posture. Gently tilting the pelvis backward and forward in a rocking motion during labour can help to lessen pain and assist the baby to descend the birth canal.

14   Reclining Stretches

Caution

These exercises are all done in the reclining position which most women find very relaxing and enjoyable in pregnancy. If, however, you are not comfortable lying flat on your back, then leave out these stretches. They are not intended for labour.

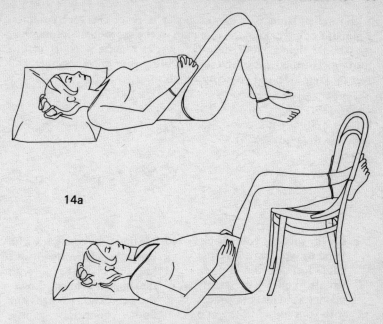

14a

14a. Lie down on your back with knees bent or your calves up on a chair. Place your hands on your belly. Close your eyes and be aware of your breathing. Then lie very still and breathe deeply for a few minutes – feel your belly rise as you inhale and fall as you exhale.

14b

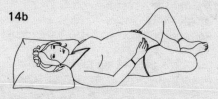

14b. Let your knees drop apart, bring the soles of your feet together as close to your body as possible. Try to keep your lower back flat on the ground. Continue breathing deeply. This stretch opens and relaxes the pelvis. Babies and young children who still have their natural flexibility can sleep quite comfortably in this position. This is a good stretch to do in bed just before falling asleep or awakening.

If you suffer from pain in the lower back or the very common complaint of pregnancy, sciatic pain in the sacro-illiac joints, then you should tighten your buttock muscles especially while in this position. To come out of the stretch, bring your knees together, roll over on your side and come up on all fours.

14c
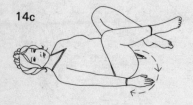

14d
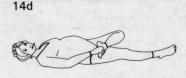

14c. Lie down on your back. Bending your knees, cross your feet at the ankles. Rotate your legs gently making a circular movement with your hips. Make 2 or 3 circles and then change directions. In this way you can massage your lower back. This is very useful and relaxing and relieves fatigue, particularly in the later months of pregnancy.

14d. Lie down on your back with legs extended. Bend one knee and clasp the foot with the opposite hand. Lower the bent knee towards the floor, bouncing gently. Repeat several times and then change to the other foot. This exercise is particularly helpful in relieving pain in the sacro-illiac joint.

14e
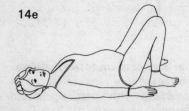

14f
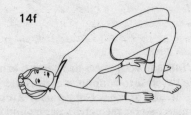

14e. and f. Lie flat on your back, bend your knees and bring your feet up towards your buttocks. Be aware of how your back contacts the floor. Tuck in your pelvis, pressing your lower back into the floor. Tighten your buttock muscles and then, keeping them tight, raise your pelvis so that your spine lifts up as far as your shoulder blades. Hold for a second and then exhale as you come down. Repeat 3 or 4 times.

How you feel   You should feel the stretch in your thighs.

How you benefit   This exercise strengthens the buttock muscles, giving support to your lower back. It corrects the tilt of the pelvis and also extends the front of the spine, opening the front of your body in a way that is completely safe for pregnancy. This stretch will help or prevent backache or sacro-illiac pain.

15   Twist

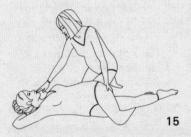

Work with a partner, if possible. Lie down on your back. Clasp your hands behind your head. Bend your knees and cross your legs, tucking one foot behind your calf – or else simply bend your knees. Twist your body gently so that your upper knee goes towards the ground.

15

Your partner should kneel beside you and hold down your elbow with one hand, gently exerting pressure in the middle of your lower back to increase the stretch. Hold for a minute or two, breathing deeply, and then change to the other side.

How you feel   You should feel this stretch in the muscles that support your breasts above your armpit. You should also feel a pleasant stretching sensation along the side of your trunk.

How you benefit   This stretch is a spinal twist and lubricates the joints between the vertebrae and opens your chest.

It also relaxes the muscles which support your breasts and the intercostal muscles between your ribs.

It releases the lower back and stretches parts of your body like your sides in a completely non-strenuous safe way for pregnancy.

This stretch will help or prevent lower back and sacro-illiac pain.

16 Resting

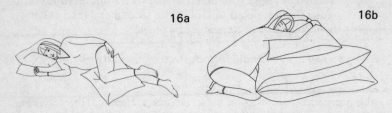

16a   16b

It is advisable to rest for at least 10 minutes after a stretch session. Turn over on your side. Place a pillow under your head. Extend your bottom leg and bend your top leg placing a pillow under your knee.

This is a resting position and is also very comfortable for sleep.

Alternatively, kneel comfortably on the floor or on your bed, with knees apart, leaning on a large floor cushion or pile of cushions so that your whole body is supported and you can rest. This is another good resting position for pregnancy and is particularly useful during labour.

Your Daily Practice

To get the most benefit from the stretches try to practise some (if not all) of them every day. The essential exercises are:

Butterfly (2)
Japanese sitting (3)
Legs apart on the wall (4)
Squatting (11)

Do these every day as a basic minimum adding others which are helpful to you.

If you intend to do them all then follow as a sequence from 1 to 16.

3
The Facts of Birth

Your uterus lies deep inside your abdominal cavity, between the bladder in front and the rectum behind. These are known as the pelvic organs. Your abdominal cavity extends from your diaphragm, beneath your lungs, to the muscles of the floor of your pelvis.

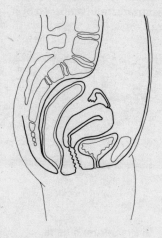

The pelvic organs

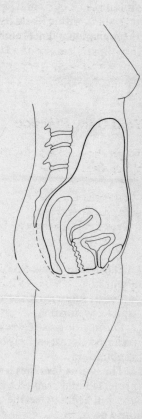

The abdominal cavity

Before pregnancy your uterus is a small, hollow muscular organ, shaped like an inverted pear, measuring roughly 3 in. × 2 in. × 1 in.

Extending to each side from the top part or *fundus* are two narrow canals, the Fallopian tubes, which end in finger-like projections called *fimbria* which surround your ovaries on either side and draw up the ripe *ovum* after you ovulate.

The lower part or mouth of the uterus is called the *cervix* which projects into the vagina and will open up during labour to allow your child to be born. During pregnancy your cervix is closed and the narrow opening is sealed with a mucous plug. The cervix is about 1½ in. long.

The uterus is the principal organ involved in pregnancy and childbirth. Your child is conceived in one of its Fallopian tubes, implanted within its cavity and at the appropriate time is expelled by it through your vagina into the outside world.

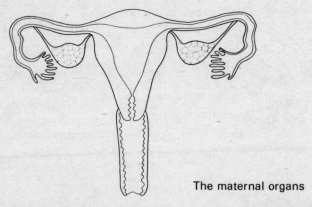

The maternal organs

During the 40 weeks of pregnancy, your uterus increases in size to about 12 in. × 9 in. × 9 in. Its weight increases from 100 grams to 1,000 grams at full term and the amount of fluid it contains grows from ¼ tspn to 5½ litres.

During the first 16 weeks of pregnancy the expansion of your uterus is caused almost entirely by the growth of its tissues owing to hormonal stimulation.

The uterus becomes a thick-walled organ, circular in shape and is protected and cradled by the bones of your pelvis. Around this time you will begin to feel the 'quickening' movements of your child within the womb.

From the 20th week growth almost ceases and the uterus then expands because the muscle fibres are stretched by the growing child.

The walls of the uterus become thinner and in the latter half of the pregnancy you can feel your child's body quite easily from outside. Your uterus becomes more oval in shape and moves up into your abdomen as your child grows.

As it enlarges its position changes. At 12 weeks the fundus is just above your pelvic inlet. At 16 weeks its upper end is nearly halfway to your navel, which it reaches at the 18th week. At 36 weeks the top part of your uterus is lying just below your diaphragm, at the level of the lower end of your breastbone. During the last few weeks it drops a little lower as your baby settles into position for birth.

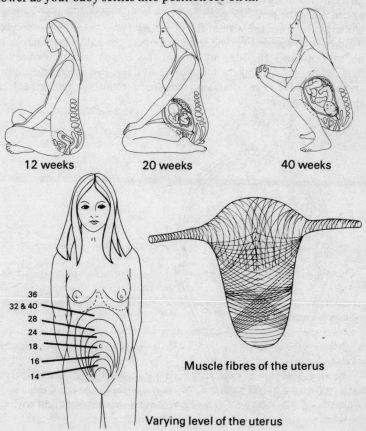

12 weeks   20 weeks   40 weeks

36
32 & 40
28
24
18
16
14

Muscle fibres of the uterus

Varying level of the uterus

Your uterus is a hollow muscular organ which consists of a network of muscle fibres and bundles running in all directions, longitudinal, oblique and circular.

During pregnancy your baby lies within the uterus connected from his navel by the umbilical cord to the placenta, which is attached to the wall of your uterus and draws nourishment for your child from your bloodstream and simultaneously passes waste products back to you. The umbilical cord is made up of three intertwined blood vessels, two veins carrying blood from the baby back to the placenta and one artery which carries blood from the placenta to the baby.

Your baby has an independent blood circulation system which flows all round the body through the umbilical cord to the placenta and back again. After the birth the placenta is no longer needed and in a while will separate from the wall of the uterus and pass through the cervix. Your baby's placenta, for indeed it belongs to the baby in the uterus, is about one-third the size of your baby and is surrounded by a membrane. It looks like a large piece of liver. If it is examined and spread out one can see that it is a network of blood vessels, rather like the roots of a tree.

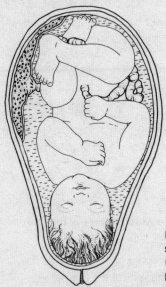

Baby at term in the womb surrounded by waters and membranes with cord and placenta

A bag of membranes surrounds your baby, the placenta and cord and also contains approximately 5½ litres of amniotic fluid – the waters within which your baby lies. These waters protect your baby from shock or infection and are constantly being replenished by your body.

At full term, at the end of pregnancy, the main function of your uterus is to evacuate its contents. During labour the uterus will contract at regular intervals and gradually open up at its base (the cervix) to allow your baby to pass through. Once it has opened it will contract powerfully to expel your baby and the placenta, the bag of membranes and all its contents. (Placenta and membranes are called the 'afterbirth'.) In the hours and weeks after the birth your uterus will continue to contract rhythmically, stimulated by hormones.

Your baby, sucking on the breast, will stimulate the release of these contracting hormones. The uterus will gradually shrink back to its original shape and size and will expel all the blood-rich lining which was used to nourish your baby. By the end of the 6th week after birth your uterus will be back to normal and will have completed its task.

4
Labour

For the sake of convenience labour can be described in three stages: the dilation of the cervix and opening of the uterus is referred to as the first stage of labour; the expulsive stage – when your child is born – is known as the second stage of labour, and the delivery of the placenta and membranes is the third stage of labour.

In the last few weeks before labour starts you will begin to feel your uterus contracting. These pre-labour practice contractions are usually painless. You will probably feel your uterus tighten and go hard – this tightening can last for fifteen minutes or longer.

'For the last two weeks of my pregnancy I had contractions, some very strong but after a few hours they would stop.'

Any time within the last six weeks of pregnancy your baby's head will probably 'engage' in the pelvic inlet, ready for birth. You might feel some strong contractions when this happens. Some women experience frequent mild contractions a day or so before going into labour. These can start up for a few hours and then cease and are known as pre-labour. It is important to expect the possibility of a pre-labour. If you are doubtful as to whether your contractions are the real thing – probably they are not!

The big question is – *how will you know when labour is starting?*

'It was a beautiful sunny morning and Jane suggested that Ismail and I go for a walk. We took a stroll round the block, stopping every few minutes as I squatted on the pavement through a contraction, whilst Ismail, squatting besides me, massaged my lower back. The milkman must have thought we'd gone mad.'

Officially labour starts when your cervix begins to dilate, however, it can start in different ways:

1   It may start with a show, which is a discharge of pinkish-red mucous or blood, the plug which sealed your cervical opening during pregnancy. This show can come away just before labour starts or during the first stage.

'Mild contractions started about twelve hours after the "show" at five minute intervals.'

2   Sometimes the first thing to happen is the breaking of the membranes or leaking of the waters. It may come as a huge gush of amniotic fluid or a slow leaking of the water in front of the baby, known as the fore-waters. This, too, may not happen until well on in the first stage and can happen twenty-four hours or so before labour actually begins.

'I felt a "pop" and warm waters flooded out of me. I felt instantly wide awake and excited.' 'When I got up there was trickle of water and then a show, so I knew that truly she was on the way.'

3   You could feel a persistent, dull backache which may be the contractions of your uterus.

4   You could have diarrhoea as your bowels have a natural tendency to empty before labour starts.

5   You may feel very shivery and shaky. This is your body's way of letting out tension and often happens at the start of labour or at any point during the labour. The best thing to do is just let it happen until it passes, breathing deeply and perhaps having your back or feet massaged.

6   The most common sign that labour has started are contractions. These will be somewhat stronger than the pre-labour contractions. They might feel similar to period pains in the lower abdomen or else you may feel them in your lower back or inner thighs.

'I became slowly aware of that familiar tightening and mild cramp in my abdomen. As I had been in a sound sleep until that point I didn't immediately realise things had begun, but as I continued to experience these pains at five-minute intervals, more or less, it was soon obvious that baby was trying to tell us something.'

The first contractions can feel quite uncomfortable or may be so mild that you can sleep through them or are unaware of them.

Basically, contractions are experienced very differently by different women, or even by the same woman in different labours. They may be mild or strong when they start. They may come every half an hour or every ten minutes or perhaps at quite irregular intervals. Your uterus will begin to contract and tighten – thinning and drawing up the cervix and then slowly opening at its base. Each contraction comes on like a wave – starting out, building up to a peak and tailing off. There will then be a rest period before the next one starts. It helps to think of waves breaking on the shore.

Some women describe contractions as 'rushes' of energy. Anyhow, the contraction is at its strongest at the peak and can be painful at this point.

'The contractions were still very mild and 10 mins apart, when I arrived at the hospital. The nursing staff were reluctant to admit me as they said I appeared to be so calm they weren't even sure I was in labour.

'I was walking about and squatting and when I was next examined 30 minutes later, they seemed to be amazed that I was progressing so quickly. The contractions were now 5 minutes apart and quite strong and I found that by leaning forward against the wall and also kneeling on all fours on the floor I got a lot of relief.'

As the labour progresses the contractions become more frequent and more intense with shorter gaps between them.

By the time you are in well established labour the contractions will be really intense and you will need to give them all your attention.

'The contractions became a lot more demanding of me, and I mostly sat upright on the edge of my bed, leaning forward on a chair back, as I concentrated on deep "belly" breathing.'

'I started getting pains, rather like bad period pains. They came every ten minutes and I found that by breathing deeply through them I could easily cope with them. Between the pains I kept myself active, doing things around the house.'

The Sensations of Labour

Birth is a very special event in your sexual life as a woman. It is a time when you are transformed – you are becoming a mother, giving birth to another human being. During labour your womb will open up completely and you will also experience a change in your normal consciousness.

In the hours of labour you will want to withdraw from the normal day to day level of things and your attention will naturally turn inwards, as if the whole world contracts to what is happening within your body. In your mind – time takes on a fresh dimension – hours can pass in what seems like minutes – it is like being in another world.

'I felt outside of time.'

'From then onwards I was centred on my body, unaware of what was going on around me.'

This great opening of the womb happens only once or a few times in your life. It is a very deep emotional experience which involves a regression to your most basic and primitive feelings – as if everything you have ever been through is part of the present time. There is perhaps an unconscious remembrance of once being in the womb yourself, of being born, of being a very small child yet at the same time the dawning of yourself as a mother and a very intimate communion between you and your body and your child within.

Your womb is the seat of your deepest feelings. In the same way that you need to sink deeply into your inner feelings when you experience full sexual orgasm, you need to respond instinctively to the urges and messages of your body when you are in labour and about to give birth.

In a way you need to lose control, to surrender and trust in the birth process which takes place automatically. You need to let go of your mind, of everything that you know and just let it happen. This is a time to turn inwards, to abandon oneself to the unknown, not to think ahead of what is to come, just to take it moment by moment and let the natural involuntary rhythms of your body take over.

'It's easy if you can surrender to the birth force as it passes through you. If you relax you float, if you struggle and fight you sink.'

You will probably experience many intense feelings of every kind, from agony to ecstasy, despair and weakness to courage and strength, from exhaustion to incredible energy and power. You are also likely to experience some nausea. Some women never do, while others experience a lot during labour. This is nothing to be afraid of and in fact if you allow yourself to retch or vomit you will have immediate relief and this can help you to free yourself of tension and anxiety. Birth is a great emptying – and it is not surprising that your stomach and bowels tend to empty themselves of their contents at this time.

'Between those first contractions I went to the loo frequently and my baby seemed intent on a full and natural evacuation process. A few minutes later I was sick and then felt fine and ready to cope with the contractions.'

Life-giving Pain

The pain of childbirth has a bad reputation, there is no doubt about it – as any experienced mother will tell you – giving birth is painful.

It is certainly realistic to expect pain even if, in the end, you are one of the lucky few who doesn't feel any – and there are some.

Most women experience pain at the peak of contractions. The pains are acute rather than throbbing and insistent and do not generally last in between contractions. Often a very strong contraction is followed by a milder one. The pain is not the same as the pain of injury. Many women describe it as positive or life-giving pain and experience equal pleasure between contractions.

One of the main causes of unnecessary pain in childbirth is the use of the reclining position. Even if you are propped up by pillows you are like a stranded beetle – completely helpless – and the contractions of your uterus will hurt more. Other postures such as kneeling forward, standing, squatting, or sitting upright actually relieve the pain and help you to tune in to what is happening inside you. You need the freedom to use your whole body to discover how to make yourself comfortable.

'I felt incredibly uncomfortable whenever I lay down and being in an upright position was basically the only way I could fully concentrate on trying to relax and keep up the deep breathing.'

'I found small movements helpful – at one point I found I was almost dancing. Leaning against anything hard was impossible for me and lying on my back was the worst thing of all.'

Often it is the wrong kind of environment and atmosphere that causes extra pain.

During pregnancy and labour your body produces hormones called endorphines, which are natural painkillers that relax you and reduce pain. Another hormone secreted by your body is oxytocin which stimulates the contractions and the birth process. However, the secretion of these hormones is deeply connected with your emotions. For your body to produce them you need to be in a conducive, intimate environment where you feel secure and uninhibited and are free to be yourself. The presence of other unnecessary people in the room or someone you do not feel relaxed with can inhibit these secretions.

'The positions had left me feeling very uninhibited and because I was at home I felt very safe and comfortable. I moaned and groaned and released the power that way too – it felt wonderful. I was an intuitive instrument for the birth – Toby was coming and my body just opened up.'

A feeling of being watched can make you tense up. These are vital considerations when choosing the attendants and place of birth. It is important for you to feel trust and confidence in the people who are helping you and to have the comfort and support of your husband or someone close to you in labour.

'With constant encouragement from my husband and the midwife I felt spurred on to my goal. Ismail said afterwards that he was glad that he could help me – like bringing me back to my deep breathing whenever I lost control of it.'

We have spoken already about the change of consciousness in the first stage of labour. It is very helpful to be in a semi-dark environment at this time where there is the minimum of unnecessary sensory stimulation. Soft soothing music can help you as well as your attendants! To be able to immerse yourself in water is one of the most effective ways of relieving pain in labour. The use of a pool is ideal, otherwise have a warm bath or a shower. If you feel stuck or inhibited then try taking a bath.

'The bath was a big help and I found myself rotating my hips and massaging my tummy. I had a mental picture then of stroking and comforting the baby inside me through its ordeal. We were both, after all, in the same boat!'

There is a definite correlation between anxiety, fear and pain. When you are afraid or cold or over-excited your body secretes adrenalin which inhibits the birth process. Your muscles tense up, your breathing becomes shallow and generally you are running away from what is happening inside you. This increases the pain. As soon as you relax and go with it the pain lessens.

Good preparation of body and mind during pregnancy helps you to approach birth with confidence. Stretching during pregnancy will ensure that you are at your physical best for birth and enables you to make friends with your pain, and to shed some of it before the day of the birth. Meditation on your breath and your inner self will teach you to still your mind and to surrender to the powerful sensations inside you.

The size and shape of your baby and the position in which she is lying will make a difference to the pain you feel. (See chapter 7; unusual presentations.)

We all have differing abilities to tolerate pain. It is a very subjective experience and no two labours are alike. Some women will talk of unexpected depths of pain during labour while others will say they couldn't really call it pain at all.

'The pain was worse than I had imagined – it was much fiercer – I felt I was being taken up by a giant hand and shaken over a raging black sea but just when I thought I was going to drown I would be

pulled back by the eyes of my friend who had been through the experience already and knew something of what I was going through.'

'I found the birth a marvellous experience – not at all painful only uncomfortable. It was marvellous being able to move about and remain upright. I felt in control most of the time.'

When birth is active, when the environment is conducive, and when the attendants are skilful, sensitive and considerate, the pain is certainly much more tolerable. I have noticed that in these ideal circumstances very few women need or ask for pain-relieving drugs although these are usually easily available.

It is always wise, though, when approaching such an unknown adventure, to keep an open mind. If you find the pain intolerable there is no need to feel any guilt about making use of the pain-killing drugs available. These do, however, enter the bloodstream of your baby, and have certain side effects which you need to consider carefully. Some of the effects on your baby can be harmful, so do find out as much as you can about the drugs available – their pros and cons and how to make the best use of them. (See chapter 7.) There are homoeopathic remedies which do not have harmful effects (see chapter 9).

Time and time again I have heard mothers say, 'Even though it was painful, it was worth it!' Many women say that the moment of birth was like the greatest orgasm they have ever experienced. Women talk of great ecstasy and bliss, of the deepest feelings of joy and love. It is important to realise that the pain involved is only part of the great variety of intense feelings one experiences. If one cuts out the pain one generally cuts out, to some extent, the other feelings, too.

'What a sense of completion, relief, gratefulness and joy filled me. Similar feelings were shared by my husband and tears were running down his face.'

The greatest advantage of being able to accept and tolerate the pain, and allowing nature to take its course, without disturbing the whole process, is a healthy, undamaged and vigorous baby at the end of the day, and a good beginning to the relationship between you.

'This birth I found so different from that of my first baby. Then, I had been encouraged to have pethidine and I found that this made me very sleepy – not at all in control. This time, having had no drugs I remained alert and felt very much in touch with my body although I do think that the pain was more acute.'

The First Stage of Labour

Before labour begins, your baby lies within the uterus with his or her head resting on the pelvic brim ready to be born. The cervix or mouth of the uterus is tightly closed and sealed by a mucous plug. The membranes surrounding your baby are intact and contain the waters in which the baby floats. Before labour starts the cervix is about $1\frac{1}{2}$ in. thick, and in the week before the birth it will soften and become ripe.

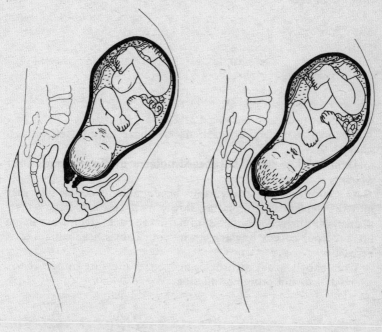

Baby in the womb at term   The cervix thinned

What happens to your baby

Before the onset of labour your baby's head engages in the pelvic brim. The widest diameter of his or her head, from the crown to the

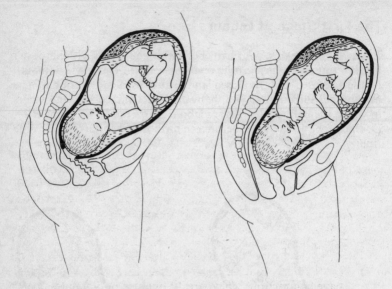

The early first stage   The late first stage

forehead, will be lying in the widest diameter of your pelvic inlet which is from side to side.

As your uterus dilates the baby's head gradually descends further into the pelvic cavity, rotating slowly as it descends. The widest diameter of the pelvic outlet is from front to back – from your pubic bone to your coccyx – which is why your baby's head rotates as it descends.

Your baby's head, as it descends, exerts pressure on the cervix which assists and promotes dilation.

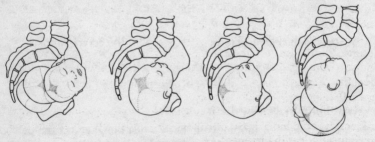

The descent of the baby's head

What happens to you

When labour starts the early contractions will draw up the cervix, so that it thins out and becomes ready to open up. Sometimes this thinning takes place in the days before labour actually begins – particularly with second and subsequent babies. You may have a pre-labour in the twenty-four hours or so preceding the birth, with mild contractions that stop and start periodically. Eventually the contractions will begin to take on a regular rhythm.

The classic labour starts with regular contractions 20–30 minutes apart and 20–30 seconds long. After some time, as your cervix dilates, they progress to 15 minutes apart (30–35 seconds long), then 10 minutes apart (35–40 seconds long), 5 minutes apart (40–45 seconds long), 3 minutes apart (45–50 seconds long), until finally, at the end of the first stage, when the cervix is almost fully open, the contractions are 60–90 seconds long with half a minute between them.

However, very few women have such a classic labour and there is great variety in the patterns and rhythms that can occur. Some women have contractions which are 10 minutes or 5 minutes apart throughout.

The length of the first stage varies enormously, the shortest being about half an hour and the longest can be 2 or 3 days with contractions stopping at times. However, the average length of the first stage for a first birth is 8–16 hours.

Whatever the rhythm of your labour, the contractions will become more powerful, longer and closer together as your cervix progressively opens and dilates from 0–10 cm (full dilation is 10 cm).

You or your midwife can feel the cervix dilating by vaginal examination, which is why you often hear the expression, 4 or 5 fingers dilated.

As you approach full dilation the contractions are at their most intense and you are nearing the peak of the labour.

In modern hospitals they are reluctant to allow a labour to take longer than twenty-four hours and often use obstetric means of induction (a syntocin drip) to accelerate a long labour. One of the benefits of active birth is that contractions tend to be more regular and efficient and labours shorter.

Your uterus tilts forward as it contracts, therefore it will work most efficiently and have least resistance in a position where you are upright and leaning forward.

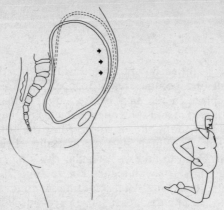

(1) The uterus tilts forward as it contracts. In the standing position there is no resistance to gravity.

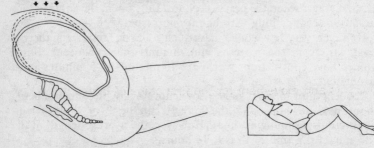

(2) In the semi-reclining position the uterus contracts against the resistance of gravity.

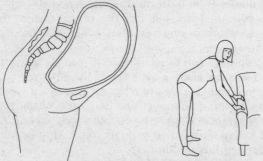

(3) By standing and leaning forward the uterus is helped to do its work with least resistance

The uterus contracting

Breathing for the first stage

Centre yourself by allowing your awareness to focus on your breathing without interfering with it, for as long as possible. When you need to, use deep belly breathing (see chapter 2, exercise 1) concentrating on the exhalation. Try to keep your shoulders relaxed by dropping them.

When the contractions become very intense you may need to make a lot of sound like groaning, moaning, humming or singing. Do not try to suppress this as it is perfectly natural to do so and can be very helpful in relieving pain. (There is research being done which reveals that making sound causes the production of hormones that act as natural pain-killers, and help to change the level of consciousness.) It is well known in various forms of meditation and religious worship that singing, or chanting, helps to still the mind and to bring one to a deeper more concentrated state of awareness.

'As the contractions increased I found myself groaning and crying out. When the pain increased and became overpowering, I still knew inside that I was in control.'

Positions and movement for the first stage of labour

In early labour it is a good idea to loosen up by doing some stretching (leave out the reclining positions).

Take a warm bath and just carry on with your usual activities until the contractions demand your full attention. If your labour starts at night try to get a little sleep, it may help you to conserve your energy for the really strong labour to come. If you can't sleep then rest in a comfortable upright position.

Arrange your room so that you have a low stool (or pile of large books) to squat on, something firm to kneel on, a soft mat or blanket to place under your knees and plenty of cushions with one or two large, firm floor cushions. A hot water bottle may be useful. The positions shown below are the basic movements which come naturally during the first stage. Use them as a guide and change positions from time to time. Try to make yourself comfortable and above all let your own instincts guide you. Allow yourself a few contractions to get used to a new position. It may help to move your pelvis rhythmically during contractions, either rocking to and fro, from side to side or in slow circles, as this will aid the dilation of your cervix, the descent of your baby and help to dissipate the pain.

'I felt the contractions so strongly that I could really only do one thing: walk, walk, walk – at quite a pace.'

Walking or standing, or 'ambulation', in labour is now recognised by experts, who have done research into the subject, to shorten labour and increase the efficiency of contractions. In the early part of the first stage try to walk about, leaning forward for contractions.

'For the first stage I began by keeping upright and walking round the delivery room then during the contraction I leant slightly forward and held onto the end of the bed, while my husband massaged my back. I moved my hips in circles during the contractions. I didn't find them at all painful only uncomfortable.'

With your body vertical the descent of the baby is helped by the downward force of gravity. Some women like to stand up throughout labour – even for delivery. Others have remarked that holding onto a rope or pole and hanging minimises the pain (there are drawings of primitive women doing the same thing). It can be helpful to put your arms around the neck of another person and hang. The supporter should keep his or her shoulders down, bend the knees slightly and tighten the buttock muscles in order to carry your weight without getting an aching back. It is important to practise this!

Many women find it comforting to be held during the contractions and have a need for the close bodily contact of another person – often another woman. Some like to stand, leaning forward onto the wall

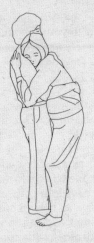

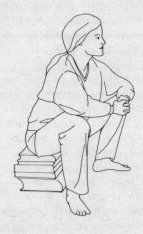

The standing position   Squatting on a low stool

during contractions and squat in between them on a low stool.

'Later in the afternoon my man and I went walking alone. I just wanted to hold him during the contractions. I felt such a strength from his energy. When I came into the house the contractions were very strong and I held Kurt round the neck and hung down. Until the final stage of my labour I had not related much to my man, finding I needed the soft quality of the women but at the end it was wonderful to have his support both mental and physical.'

Squatting is the physiological position for labour and birth. Your pelvis is at its most open, gravity is helping and contractions are at their strongest.

Use the support of another person or a stool, a pile of books or a firm cushion to make yourself as comfortable as possible.

You may squat during contractions or in between them. Squatting is very useful at any stage of labour, particularly if you wish to speed things up. Some women find this the most comfortable posture.

'I continued to squat through contractions as this position seemed most natural and comfortable to me, especially spreading my knees as wide apart as I could and squirming from side to side, all the while trying to keep my breathing slow and deep, concentrating on breathing out.'

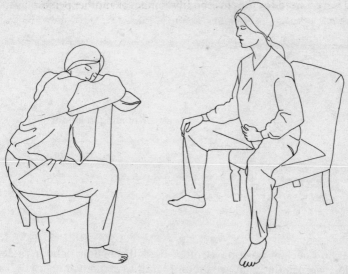

Sitting forward and backward on a chair

In these positions you have almost the same advantages as in squatting, and your trunk is supported. You can rest quite comfortably between contractions.

'I became absorbed by the contractions. I felt pain but not fear and trusted the process that was happening. I had the need to be on my own. I walked, knelt and squatted as the contractions increased, I found that the toilet seat was a very comfortable place because it supported me while leaving my pelvic floor free.'

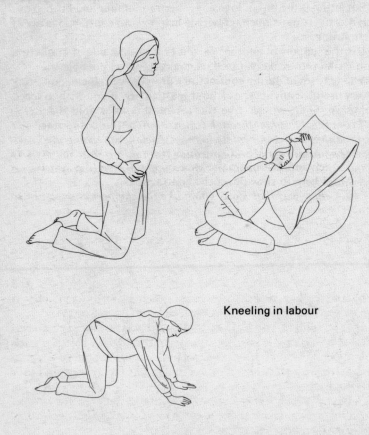

Kneeling in labour

The kneeling position is often used throughout labour, indeed most women find that as labour intensifies and advances to the last part of the first stage, say 7–10 cm dilation, kneeling is the most comfortable. You may find it helpful to move your pelvis rhythmically during contractions, either rotating or rocking.

'I went on all fours where I found a gentle rocking movement eased the pain. My boyfriend rubbed the lower part of my back almost continuously.'

The kneeling positions are very helpful if you have a 'backache labour' or if the baby is lying in a posterior position (see chapter on difficult presentations). The rhythmic rotation of the pelvis can help the baby to turn to the more usual anterior position.

You may prefer to kneel with your trunk upright or to lean forward onto a firm pile of cushions or piece of furniture. Make sure that the angle of your trunk is quite vertical to allow gravity to assist you.

'When the contractions became much stronger I moved to the beanbag. I rested against this and rotated my hips. It really did help, in fact it seemed the most natural thing to do!'

If labour is progressing rapidly you could use a more horizontal kneeling position if you wish to slow things down a little. The less vertical and more horizontal your body, the slower the contractions, as the downward force of gravity on the cervix lessens. In the case of a very sudden and fast birth, the knee-chest position (see drawing on p. 82) will help to slow down the contractions.

'All I knew was that I was going like the clappers and wanted to slow it down. I was kneeling on the floor so I put my head down onto the floor and my bottom up in the air.'

You will find that you can relax totally in between contractions in the kneeling position and the pain is more bearable. Use a foam pad in a pillow case or a folded blanket under your knees.

Kneeling is used in many religions as a position for prayer and helps one to enter a deeper level of consciousness and to surrender to the powerful energy of the contractions within your body.

Half kneeling and half squatting is a good position to use combined with kneeling and is easier than squatting. Change legs for each contraction and rock forwards and backwards towards your upper knee during contractions. This posture assists the dilation and may ease backache.

'I found the half kneeling position comfortable, in fact it was during a strong contraction in the latter position that the waters broke and I found that a great relief.'

If you wish to lie down during the first stage it is preferable to do so on your side, with your trunk well propped up by cushions, and perhaps a pillow under one knee.

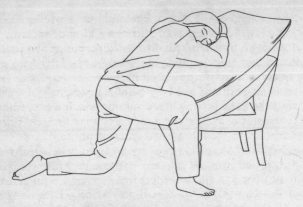

Half-kneeling, half-squatting

Transition – the end of the first stage

I once heard a midwife explain to a woman in labour that the first stage was rather like climbing a high mountain and at the end of the steep incline one reaches a very difficult craggy bit. Although the top and the view down the other side is close at hand, one can lose sight of the end and fall into despair struggling with these last difficult crags. This is an apt description of transition. It is like a bridge between the last dilating contractions and the beginning of the bearing down in the second stage. Transition can last for as little as a few seconds or as long as 2 or 3 hours. It is more common to have a long transition with a first birth.

What happens to you

Your contractions are coming fast and furious with very short intervals between them. Your cervix is probably 8–9 cm dilated, but that last cm may be very slow in disappearing. A common occurrence at this stage is what is known as an anterior lip, i.e. the front rim or lip of the cervix still needs to be taken up before the way is clear to bear down and push out your baby.

How you feel   This is not easy to describe. Most women find this the most trying part of the labour. There you are, wide open and completely vulnerable. It's too late to take anything (and very unwise). You are not yet ready to bear down, although you may begin to feel the first urges. You may be feeling desperate and irritable at one moment and then suddenly ecstatic. At this stage you can feel that you have reached the end of your tether and may forget that you are about to give birth to a baby and lose faith in everything. You are still feeling the final dilating contractions which are opening your womb to its widest, while the very different bearing down urges may be beginning. This can result in a feeling of confusion – of not knowing what is happening or where you are. In a while when the expulsive contractions are progressing the confusion will pass.

The sensations you will be feeling will be very powerful. You may feel nauseous or trembly, your head may be hot while your feet may be cold. The important thing to remember is that it will pass and that the long haul of the first stage is almost over. Most women appear to

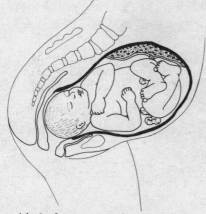

Transition

be in a kind of trance at this stage of labour – in a very deep and open state of consciousness.

'I squatted on the mattress, supported on both sides by my friend and my husband – and I had a rather short, but extremely relaxed transition period. I believe I even slept for a spell.'

'This was the most difficult part as I didn't realise I was in transition and felt I wanted to push. I was worried as this seemed far too early to want to push. I knelt forward onto the cushions. I found that eye contact with my husband was important at this stage. When I felt panic during transition my husband breathed with me to slow my breathing down. This immediately brought me back in control.'

What happens to your baby

Your baby descends a little further into the pelvic canal. The uterus has been drawn up around the baby's head so that he or she is beginning to move out of the uterus ready to be born.

Positions and movement for Transition

Once again follow your own instincts and use any position you have found helpful so far.

The kneeling position is the most popular at this stage. Use a good firm pile of cushions or else lean forward onto another person so that you can rest completely supported in the short breaks between contractions. Allow yourself to sink into a deep inner relaxation.

It is helpful to take sips of water or fruit juice, or to suck on a natural sponge (women often experience a primitive sucking reflex during labour). Bathe your face with a face cloth rinsed out in cold water to refresh yourself between contractions. You may like to sit back on your heels and stretch your arms up between contractions.

'My Mother-in-law gave me sips of warm water with a little honey added and washed my hands and face. Another thing which I found very comforting and refreshing during the whole labour was to suck upon a wet sponge.'

If you have a very long transition try changing positions from time to time. Sitting upright on the edge of the bed or on a chair, standing up, walking slowly or lying on your side – well propped up by cushions.

It may help to make more space for your baby and help your cervix to open if you try to squat a few times either during or between contractions.

Knee-chest position for an anterior lip

Your midwife will probably examine you internally at this stage to see if you are fully dilated. If she cannot feel the cervix at all you are ready to bear down and give birth to your baby. If, however, she can still feel a little rim of cervix in front of the baby's head, this is called an anterior lip. You may already be feeling the first urges to bear down, but it is probably better to wait until the lip has gone.

It is not a good idea to resist the powerful bearing down urges for long, so try the knee-chest position for a few contractions, with your head lower than your bottom.

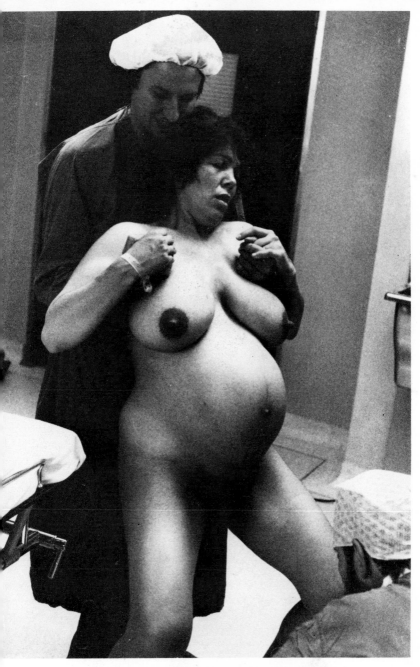

1   The second stage of labour begins. Supported squatting in a hospital setting.

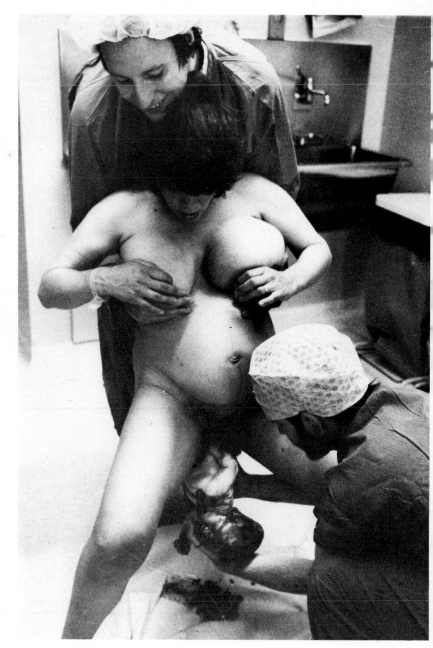

2   Both parents watch the baby being born.

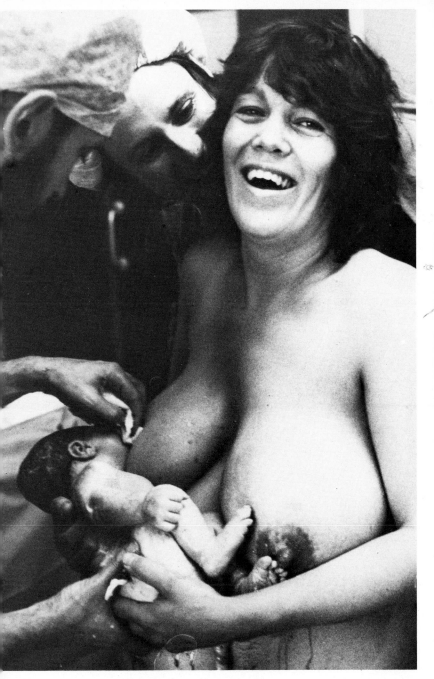

3   Moments after birth.

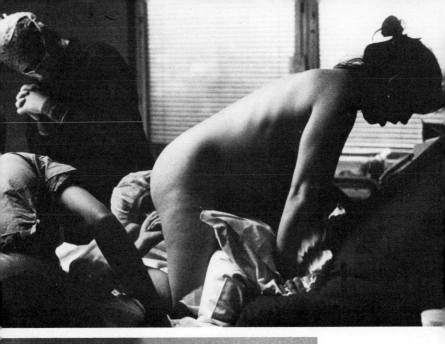

4 Birth in the kneeling position on a hospital delivery bed.

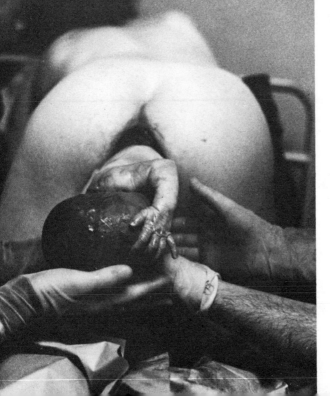

5 The baby is born.

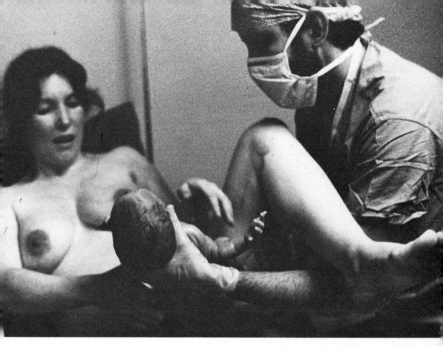

6   Mother turns to receive her baby.

7   First contact with the breast moments after birth.

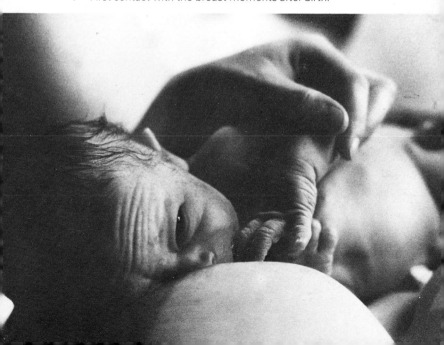

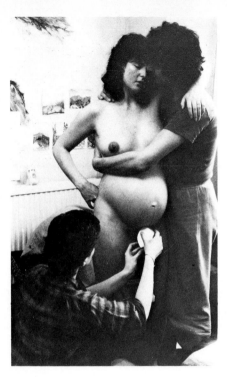

8 Between contractions the midwife checks the baby's heartbeat with a portable sonic-aid heart monitor.

9 Transition.

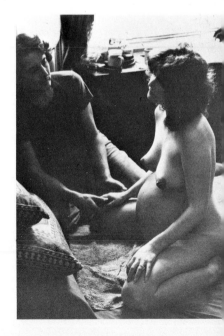

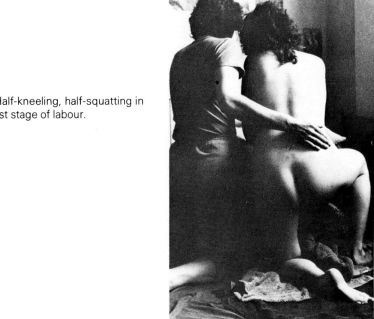

10   Half-kneeling, half-squatting in the first stage of labour.

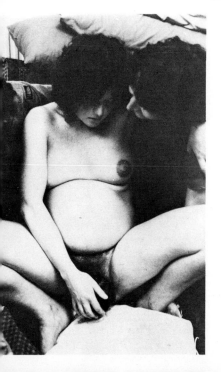

11   Supported in the squatting position the mother feels her baby's head emerge in the second stage.

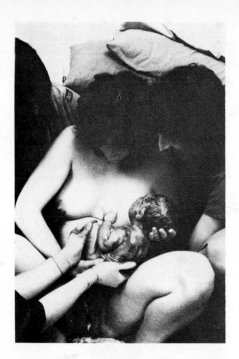

12   The baby is born.

13   The mother sits upright on a hospital delivery bed moments after an active birth. In this position she enjoys perfect contact with her baby. The umbilical cord has stopped pulsating but has not yet been cut.

Photographs:
Anthea Sieveking,
Vision International

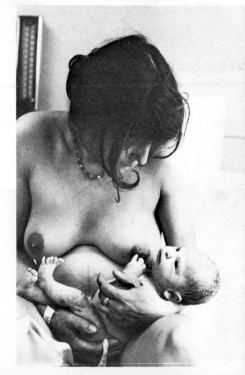

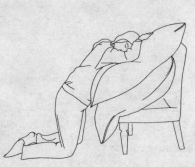

Kneeling in transition

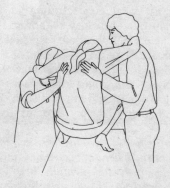

Supported squatting in transition

This position brings the baby forward and allows your cervix to retract while reducing the urge to push. Move your hips a little during contractions to assist the dilation. The lip will probably have gone after a few contractions. If the urge to bear down is very strong then try blowing out firmly when you have the urge, as if you are blowing out a candle three feet away. If you need to, ask your midwife to check if the lip has gone after four or five contractions. It is usually not necessary to stay in this position for very long.

'Billie felt an anterior lip and I went into a knee-chest position to counteract the strong pushing urge. Fortunately after only a few contractions and blowing it went and I got up.'

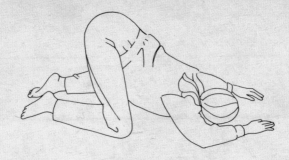

Knee-chest position

Breathing for Transition

Keep up your deep breathing as usual concentrating on the exhalation. If your breathing naturally becomes shallower then follow your own instincts. It will help you to be more relaxed if you focus your attention on the outbreath.

Some women need to make quite a lot of noise at this stage of the labour and find that it helps to relieve pain, whilst others need to be very quiet. It is most important that you should not be disturbed or distracted unnecessarily. Peace and quiet will help you to sink deeply inwards at this stage.

'The thing I found a tremendous help and relief was making a furious grunting, squealing noise at the height of each pain. It was a way of controlling myself both physically and mentally.'

'The contractions were very powerful and I began to feel extremely tired between them. I flopped forward onto two big cushions and felt as though I could sleep even for the few moments between contractions. The conservation of energy was simply wonderful, I didn't even speak when spoken to.'

The Second Stage of Labour

The second stage begins when the cervix is completely dilated and your baby's head has moved out of the uterus and into the birth canal. This stage ends with the perineum stage, or crowning, when your child is born.

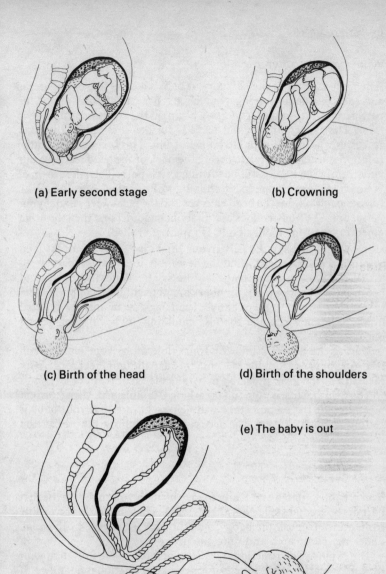

(a) Early second stage

(b) Crowning

(c) Birth of the head

(d) Birth of the shoulders

(e) The baby is out

The second stage of labour

What happens to your child

After full dilation of the cervix your baby's head is free of the uterus and the contractions bring your child's head to the middle of the pelvic canal. At this point rotation begins as the head meets the pelvic floor. Descent continues and there is further rotation as the head comes down under the pubic bone in front. This takes time, and the rotation is usually complete before the back of the head reaches your vulva, although it may still be turning as it is born. Then the crown of your child's head appears, stretching your vaginal opening. With further contractions the head emerges and the face sweeps under your perineum. The body rotates and first one shoulder and then the other emerges, until the child's body is rapidly expelled.

In passing through the pelvis your child's head has been subjected to considerable pressure. That the descent is done without damage to the head is made possible by the softness of the bones themselves and because the edges of the skull bones are not yet fused, enabling them to overlap slightly. Your baby's head may seem slightly pointed in shape after birth due to this 'moulding', but will soon round out.

During the delivery, and for some time after, your child is still receiving oxygen from the placenta through the umbilical cord. After the birth of the head the baby may take his first breath of air, but it will be a short while before full breathing is established. Using upright positions for the second stage will help to ensure that your baby is getting as much oxygen as he needs and will minimise the pressure on his or her head.

What happens to you

You are fully dilated and ready to give birth to your baby. In the first part of the second stage your uterus will begin to contract powerfully from above to push the baby down through the curved birth canal, under the pubic arch and onto the pelvic floor.

The expulsive contractions may start before you are fully dilated or they may begin 5–10 minutes, or longer, after dilation is complete. If you have a gap where nothing happens make the most of it and rest, in readiness for the birth. If you have had a long transition your uterus may need to rest. There are great variations in the length of the second stage in different women, ranging between two and three minutes and as many hours.

'My cervix was fully dilated but my body did not feel quite ready to push. It was resting, getting ready for the final stage. This lasted over an hour.'

How you feel These contractions feel quite different from the previous ones, the intervals between them are generally longer. Even if you have felt very tired at the end of the first stage, a new rush of very powerful energy often comes to help you give birth to your baby. Women describe these contractions as huge tidal waves of sensation throughout the whole body.

'I wasn't sure what I was supposed to feel until suddenly I got a terrific urge to push – which felt quite different to anything so far. With perfect timing, the doctor arrived. The second stage took ½ hour but I had no sense of time. It seemed very quick to me.'

There is usually a tremendous urge to bear down. (Although this is not the case for all women.) If you do not resist or run away from these feelings, but go along with them, they can be extremely enjoyable. The urge to bear down is very powerful and the muscular effort is often pleasant. Pressure at this stage builds up enormously and any resistance to the expulsive effort causes discomfort and pain.

Try to allow the natural rhythm to lead you, let your body be your guide and your uterus will take care of the rest.

'Nature took over – my whole body helped automatically and rhythmically in the enormous effort of pushing out a baby. I felt his head, shoulders and body being born.'

The crowning

Your baby's head will extend backwards as it descends the birth canal. Finally the crown of the baby's head will begin to show through your vagina. Feel his or her head with your hand as it descends. It is a memorable feeling and will help you to know exactly what is happening.

'I instinctively put my hand down to feel for the baby's head and there it was, crowning.'

To be born your child will have to pass through your pelvic floor. In view of its action in childbirth, the pelvic floor can be regarded as consisting of two parts; the front pubic part and the back sacral part which is attached to your buttock bones, coccyx and sacrum. As your baby comes through, the pubic area is pulled inwards and the sacral part is pushed backwards to make room for his head and body.

The pubic part has comparatively few voluntary muscles joining it to your pubic bones, whereas the sacral part has almost 90 per cent of all the pelvic floor muscles connected to it. This part of the pelvic floor is known as the perineum.

To be free to move backwards when the baby is born, the sacral area of your pelvic floor (or perineum) must be in a passive state of relaxation. The position of your body at this stage is all important. If you are lying on your back your sacrum is not free to move backwards, and the back sacral part of your pelvic floor is not in a passive relaxed state. This forces your child's head to press forward towards the bony subpubic arch instead of backwards towards your sacrum and coccyx, which are mobile and extendable. But if you are squatting, kneeling or standing, the position of your pelvis is altered, and your sacrum and coccyx are extended back. Your back sacral area will be relaxed if your child's head presses against it, allowing as much give as possible. The crowning ends with the birth of the baby.

You may have one contraction when your baby's head is born and then a pause before the next contraction when the rest of the body emerges. Once the head is born, your baby will turn and first one shoulder and then another will appear and finally the whole body will slip out.

How you feel   At this stage the sensations one feels are very intense – a unique mixture of pain and ecstasy. At the end of the crowning, when the head is about to be born and the perineal tissues stretch to their maximum, there can be a feeling of acute stretching and burning – similar to how it feels when you pull at the corners of your mouth with your fingers – mingled with the total body sensation of the contractions. However, as soon as the head (which is the widest part of the baby's body) is born there is a tremendous feeling of relief. Sometimes, if the baby is broad shouldered, one can feel further stretching, as first one shoulder and then another is born, but as your baby's body slithers out into the world the sensations are usually very pleasurable and often described as totally orgasmic.

'That was the only pushing I did, the baby came out so gradually and easy without any pushing from me. I felt a burning sensation in my perineum as he was being born and on checking I didn't even have a tear.'

'I felt an incredible presence in the room and feelings were high. The pain was almost unbearable yet now the overpowering urge to bear down was there. It was one of the most powerful bodily

sensations I think I've ever had and soon I saw her head in the mirror, a patch of thick black hair. With an extraordinary release of energy her head came out but the energy to push was so strong that immediately after her whole body shot out. The emotion was of the utmost release and joy and wonder and thankfulness. Words cannot express that feeling at the moment of birth. I wanted to cry and shout for joy.'

Breathing for the Second Stage

There is usually no need to control your breathing in the second stage of labour if you are in an upright, squatting or kneeling position.

Breathe deeply in the usual way as you feel the contraction coming on – concentrating on the outbreath and giving way to the powerful messages coming from inside your body. There is a distinctive birth cry which is natural and instinctive during the second stage, particularly as the baby is actually being born. It is unwise to resist these natural urges to cry out as they are nature's way of assisting you to give birth.

Do not tense up against the contractions of your uterus as this can be very painful, just let yourself go and release your pelvic floor, let your breath go and let the sound go as you allow your baby to be born. Women often say that when they screamed during the second stage they felt no pain at all.

You will probably feel very powerful bearing-down urges and an uncontrollable desire to push downwards at the peak of the contraction as your uterus presses down to expel your baby. Follow the natural urges of your body. Don't hold your breath as this diminishes the supply of oxygen going to you and your baby at a time when it is critical that he should have enough.

At the crowning of your baby's head try not to push too hard as this will lessen the chances of a perineal tear. Some women find it helpful to pant as the head is born, while others prefer to abandon themselves completely at this moment.

'I squatted on the bed supported by the midwife and my husband, and felt my baby emerging. I put my arms under me and feeling the head I let out an earthly primitive moan, letting the baby slide into my hand. She was warm, creamy, smoother and softer than anything I had ever touched.'

If the second stage is difficult – for instance, if you have a very large baby, an unusual presentation or a very slow second stage – you may find it helpful to bear down actively during the contraction. Wait until the contraction begins and then take in a good breath and as you exhale direct your energy downwards, pressing down inside with your diaphragm muscle in exactly the same way you would do to help yourself when defecating. Do not hold your breath. Sometimes lots of little pushes work better than one long one. Practise this gently in the squatting position in case you need to use it in labour.

Above all, in the second stage, keep in harmony with the rhythmic sensations you are feeling. Allow them to lead you. Surrender to what your body is telling you.

'During the 1½ hours of second stage, I was squatting on the floor almost the whole time, occasionally standing. I felt as comfortable as I could imagine being in labour and the position, being well supported, enabled me to control my breathing and work with the expulsive contractions as much as possible. I also had a really good view of the emerging head, in a mirror propped up in front of me. I gave birth to the baby in the same squatting position.'

Positions for the Second Stage

Your posture makes all the difference to the length and efficiency of the second stage. You will make your child's descent easier if you position your pelvis at its widest and use vertical, upright positions which allow gravity to help in the safe delivery of your child.

Try this

Squat down on your toes. Breathe in and tighten your pelvic floor, hold for a second and then let go slowly as you breathe out. Repeat several times.

Now try the same thing lying down in the reclining position with a pillow under your head. You will probably find that in this position the movement of your perineum is much weaker and more effort is needed on your part to let go of the pelvic floor muscles.

Try it again squatting and compare the difference when gravity helps the pelvic floor to relax.

The fit between your child's head and your pelvis is so exact that the smallest increase in the size of your pelvis is significant.

Try this
Squat down on your toes and spread your knees apart. Close your eyes and be aware of the opening of your pelvis. In fact, it is open at its widest in this position and your sacrum and coccyx are free to move if your child was passing through your pelvic outlet.

Now try the semi-reclining position. Place your hand under your back and feel how the whole weight of your body, your uterus and baby is lying on your sacrum which is closed to its maximum in this position. (Research suggests that you are losing a significant percentage of the possible opening.)

The weight of your uterus also presses down on the large internal blood vessels in your abdomen in this reclining position, which reduces the supply of oxygen going to your baby and is the best way to induce foetal distress.

Your uterus tilts forward when it contracts. In this position it must work against the downward force of gravity. This will make contractions more painful and less efficient.

'On one occasion I was lying on my back to enable Jane to examine me. Unfortunately I had a contraction whilst in this position. It was extremely painful and I would not like to repeat that experience.'

Your coccyx is designed to move out of the way as your baby's head descends to make more room – all the more reason not to sit on it! (It can lead to dislocation of the coccyx which can be extremely painful for months after the birth.)

These are some of the reasons why women, who have the freedom to choose their own position for delivery, rarely choose the semi-reclining one much less to lie down on their backs! (For instance, in one year at Pithiviers only 2 out of 1,000 chose to lie down.)

Each position has certain advantages. You will find out instinctively which position is best for you at the time. Try them out with your partner in the weeks before the birth so your body will know all the possibilities. Also, sometimes, the room and circumstances in which you give birth will dictate the position you choose. Ideally the room should contain little furniture so that you can freely discover the right posture. However, it is possible to use natural birth positions either on a bed or on the floor. (See chapter 7, Active birth at home or in hospital.) Unless the second stage is very short it is likely that you will change positions – standing and squatting, or squatting and kneeling, or kneeling and sitting up as your baby descends. It is helpful to have two people present to help support you.

1. Supported Squatting

The standing, supported squat is highly recommended by Michel Odent.

You stand or walk in between contractions, but as the contraction comes on your knees will bend and someone supports you from behind, holding you under your arms or at the wrists, while you let your weight go completely and surrender to the force of the contraction.

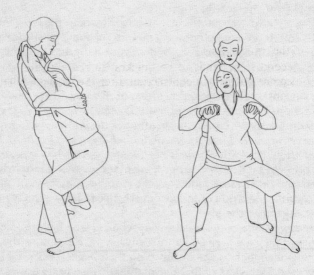

Different ways of supporting in the standing squat

After the contraction passes you move freely until the next one, when you are supported again. It is essential for the supporter to keep the shoulders down, to bend the knees slightly and to tighten the buttocks, leaning back a little so that your weight is carried against his or her pelvis. In this way even a small person can support a large and heavy woman with no strain or effort. Practise this with your partner until you have it right, as it can cause backache to your partner if done incorrectly during labour. (Your supporter should not bend forward with rising shoulders as this will put strain on the lower back.) A clean sheet and a disposable paper pad used for delivery are placed between your legs ready to receive the baby.

After the baby is born the midwife puts him or her down gently on the soft clean cloth, or pad, between your feet. The baby should be placed face down (on his belly) for a second or two. This way the fluids will drain naturally with the help of gravity, while you sit down upright on the floor and pick up the newborn infant in your arms. It is considered as extremely important not to interfere with the unfolding of this process or to disturb the mother by giving instructions.

Advantages In this position the pelvis is wide open and the verticality makes for maximum help from gravity. The upward force of the supporter's body acts as a counterbalance to the downward force of the contractions.

The second stage tends to be quickest in this posture, the baby usually comes out in one contraction after the crowning. This is a great advantage if the second stage has been long or difficult, or when there is a difficult presentation, i.e. posterior or breech, or if there is any suspicion of distress (which is less likely if the labour has been active).

The simplicity of this position allows the mother great freedom to act instinctively – to surrender to her natural urges. After the birth the simple upright sitting position facilitates an ideal bonding of mother and child (as anyone will know who has tried to put a baby to the breast while lying back).

'*With the first urges to bear down I searched for a posture to help me do so. The best one was with my husband holding me up from the back with his arms passing under mine and locked in front of me while I just let myself hang loose. It was not only a comfortable position for me but one where the sheer contact with his physical strength revived my now tired body, and it also gave us both a sense of bonding. The bearing down happened on its own and within just four pushes our baby was out: a beautiful, slippery, gurgly little girl.*'

In Odent's hospital a bath of warm water is brought for the infant and placed between the mother's legs, so that she can bathe her baby before the placenta is delivered or the umbilical cord is cut.

The loving feelings of the mother in this first contact between her and her baby – skin to skin and eye to eye – encourage the production of natural hormones which stimulate the separation of the placenta and the contraction of the uterus in the third stage.

'*He stared intently at me and then started to suck at my breast. The cord was left attaching us until it stopped pulsing and was white.*

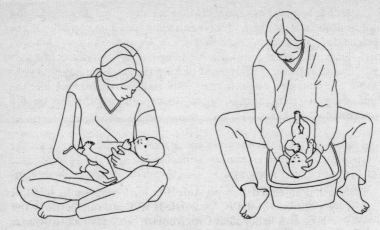

Positions for mother and newborn infant immediately after birth

There was no feeling of separation only continuation and deep joy and contentment. Everything felt right and I felt wonderful, not at all tired.'

2.   Supported squatting with two people

This position is ideal for the woman who can squat easily or has practised squatting throughout her pregnancy. The pelvis is open at its widest and gravity helps the baby to descend. During the

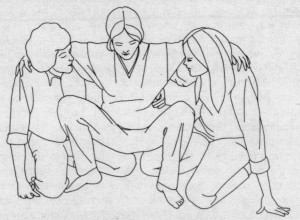

Supported squatting with two people

contraction the mother squats down on the ground and her two supporters kneel on either side of her placing one knee just under each of her buttocks. She can then put one arm around the shoulders of each supporter who in turn can put one arm each around her back. Between contractions she can stand up or kneel forward.

Advantages   In this position the mother is free to use her hands and to look down and watch her baby being born in a completely relaxed supported squat. Many women find it very helpful to use their own hands to feel the baby's head descending and to help ease the perineal tissues and deliver the baby as it is born. Some women have a strong instinct to do this themselves.

Nature has intended this position for birth because in this full squatting position the baby, unassisted, will slip out between the mother's legs and land safely in front of her, face downwards. She can then lift up the baby herself. This is also the safest position for the fluids to drain from the mother.

After the birth the mother can sit down on the floor in an upright sitting position. It is much easier for the mother to handle the baby if she is upright and for baby to find the breast.

'*For the second stage I turned and proceeded to squat, standing-up in between contractions to stretch the legs. All things considered, I felt marvellous ... confident, in control ... during this stage which lasted about ¾ hour. The obstetrician, by turning his head for a moment, missed the actual birth; Lara literally sailed out – a totally solo performance – and exercised her vocal chords immediately!*'

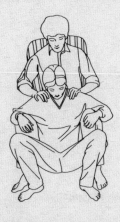

Supported squatting with partner
seated on a chair

3.   Supported squatting from behind

Here the supporter sits in a chair or on the edge of a bed and the mother squats with her body cradled between his legs and uses his knees for support. Many women find this most enjoyable and comforting as well as comfortable.

'I squatted between Ron's knees as he sat on a chair and I supported myself on his thighs with my elbows, resting my back in his lap.

'We looked in the mirror to see our baby's head emerging, then before the midwife could put her rubber gloves on all of him was born and he was placed in my arms to suckle.'

4.   Kneeling or all fours position

You simply kneel forward onto your hands and knees or onto a pile of cushions with your knees apart.

This position comes very naturally and is often used by primitive women. It is ideal if the labour and second stage are very fast as you will have more control and the baby will descend a little more slowly. It can also be very useful if the baby is in a posterior presentation as it relieves pressure on the back and you can move your hips gently to help the baby to rotate as it descends. Mothers say that this is a very simple and easy way to give birth. In between contractions you can kneel upright and stretch up your arms if you want to.

Once the baby is born and is received by the midwife she can pass the baby to you through your legs. You then sit back on your heels or upright with your baby in your arms.

Some mothers instinctively turn over after delivering in a kneeling

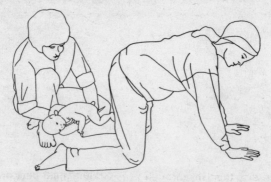

Practising the all-fours position for delivery

position. The midwife can then pass the baby to the mother under one knee as she turns. Often mothers deliver in a more upright kneeling position with one knee up. This position can be useful if the mother wishes to deliver the baby herself.

In the case of a very fast and unexpected second stage, use the knee-chest position to slow down and gain control (see chapter 9, Emergency Birth).

'When the second stage began, I knelt upright and held onto the top of the bed to push. It took no more than half an hour to push the baby out, I gave birth on all fours then without having the cord cut – I turned over and was given the baby. Wonderful! Because I was kneeling and very much in control of how fast the baby was being born, I didn't tear and so was able to walk around quite comfortably shortly after the delivery.'

5. Side lying

This can sometimes be a useful position for delivery. The sacrum is free to move but gravity will not be used to full advantage so this posture would not be sensible if the second stage was slow. However, when the baby is descending without difficulty you may be comfortable like this. Lie on your side, with your trunk well propped up by pillows and hook one arm under your knee to support your leg as the baby is born.

After the birth sit upright to hold and put your baby to the breast.

'For me, the right position was simply the one which felt right at the time. This was lying on my left side with my knees drawn to my chest and my hands drawing the opening wider and at the same time being able to have contact with the emerging head. In this way I was able to actively open my perineum with its delicate muscles and give a little tactile help.'

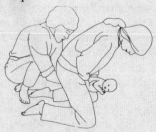

Passing the baby through
the knees

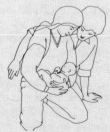

Mother sits back on her
heels with baby

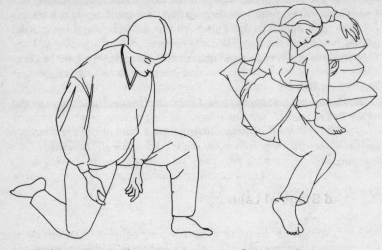

Half-kneeling, half-squatting
for delivery

Side lying for second
stage

The baby immediately after birth

As it is born and immediately after birth your baby may be a slightly
blue or greyish colour. This is perfectly normal and as soon as
breathing starts the body will become the normal pink colour. The
baby will be very slippery and moist, perhaps covered in some blood
and a white creamy substance which looks rather like butter and is
called vernix. This is important to the baby and should not be washed
off as it contains nourishing substances which are absorbed by the
baby's body and also protects the baby from the change in
temperature from your body to the room. Within a few hours this will
be absorbed by the skin. The baby may be a little wrinkled too, but
after some time the body becomes soft and round. Some babies also
have fine hairs growing on their ears or other parts of the body at
birth; these will fall out in the early weeks. The baby's head, at this
age, is quite large in proportion to the rest of the body and could be a
little pointed or 'moulded' from the birth, and the genitals are usually
a little enlarged as well.

Your baby's eyes will open very soon after the birth – perhaps even before the whole body emerges and will be awake and looking for you! All the baby's senses are acutely sensitive and alive at this stage. The skin, the ears and eyes and mouth are all receptive to any stimulation. For this first hour or two after birth the baby will be extremely alert – more so than in the hours and days to come – as she or he experiences the world, the atmosphere, breathing and sight for the first time. The lungs and digestive system begin to work independently as the baby breathes air and sucks colostrum from your breasts.

The baby will need to keep close to you, to the familiar sound of your heartbeat in the early hours, days and weeks after birth.

The Third Stage of Labour

After the birth your baby will be in your arms. The rush of emotion you will feel will cause the secretion of hormones in your body which, after a while, will cause your uterus to contract and the placenta to separate from the wall of the uterus. Nature has designed the process to take place quite automatically. As your baby comes into contact with the breast or sucks on the nipple this causes the uterus to contract strongly.

Meanwhile your baby begins to breathe independently through the lungs and after 10 to 15 minutes (if not sooner) breathing will be fully established and the umbilical cord will have stopped pulsating.

The placenta and cord continue functioning until breathing is fully established to guarantee the baby a supply of oxygen, and a means of getting rid of carbon dioxide. Particularly in the case of distress or a complication this supply of oxygen is like an insurance policy until the baby is capable of breathing by itself.

It is extremely dangerous for a newborn baby to be deprived of oxygen and can cause brain damage. It is equally dangerous for the baby to have no means of breathing out carbon dioxide. If the baby is still receiving oxygen from the placenta (if the umbilical cord is not cut prematurely) this is far less likely to occur.

A midwife once told a story of a very unusual situation, where the baby was breathing irregularly for an hour and a half. She left the cord attached and also gave the baby some oxygen occasionally until the breathing was regular. She observed that the cord continued to function for 1½ hours and then finally stopped pulsating when the baby no longer needed to breathe through the placenta. The placenta then separated and was delivered and the baby was in perfect condition.

After the cord has stopped pulsating it becomes completely flaccid and clamps itself spontaneously. It is then appropriate to cut the cord, and to separate the baby from the placenta. Many parents enjoy cutting the cord themselves – a ritual of separation which can be very satisfying.

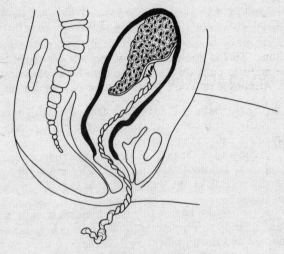

Separation of the placenta

After the cord is cut the midwife will probably feel your belly to check if the placenta has separated.

The third stage should not be rushed. Artificial stimulants (ergometrine or syntometrine) which induce contractions of the uterus are not generally necessary after active birth if the normal bonding situation has occured and if the mother has given birth in an upright position. These were invented for situations where the mother has been in labour lying down and has had an epidural, or other anaesthetic, which reduces the ability of the uterus to contract spontaneously; in the unusual case of excessive bleeding; or when mother and baby are separated at birth and the normal hormonal balance is disturbed.

After the birth the suckling of the baby at the breast will stimulate the uterus to contract and expel the placenta. This usually occurs in the first hour after the birth but can sometimes take longer. There is no need to hurry the process unless there is excessive bleeding.

You will feel the contractions coming on and could then squat in order to allow the uterus to expel the afterbirth. It is approximately one-third of the size of the baby and, unlike the baby, has no bones and is much easier to deliver. The sensations women feel as the placenta comes out are very enjoyable – it is like ending on a pleasant and healing note.

'The placenta was born half an hour later, I simply squatted over a dish and with one gentle push out it came.'

If the third stage is spontaneous there is far less likelihood of complications. This is one of the main reasons why cord-traction (where the midwife pulls on the cord to deliver the placenta) is not advisable. Although it won't hurt, it robs you of the orgasmic pleasure of delivering the placenta spontaneously.

Remember to have a look at the placenta if you want to. Hospitals usually donate placentas to cosmetic factories which use the valuable hormones to make their products.

In some societies extensive rituals surround the disposal of the afterbirth which is often regarded as having been part of the baby in the womb and having magical properties. Many animals eat the placenta – the hormones it contains help the uterus to contract and return to normal. Now and then women do the same thing (some cooking it into a stew with wine and mushrooms). Recent experiments have revealed that putting even one piece of raw placenta to the lips of the mother after birth causes the uterus to contract and can stop haemorrhages. Other people like to bury the placenta under a favourite tree – although the hospital staff will think you are crazy, while some couples take it home in a plastic bag for burial!

After the birth your doctor will examine your vagina and perineum to see if you have torn and if any stitching up is needed. If this is the case, the doctor will give you a local anaesthetic to prevent you feeling any pain and then stitch up any tears. If you do need stitching you can, if you wish, continue to hold your baby while this is being done. It is advisable to use local anaesthesia in this case as there is no danger to the baby and the stitching can be very painful without it. Even for one stitch it is worth the anaesthetic! It is not necessary to use foot stirrups if the anaesthetic is well administered as you should not feel anything.

Soothing, antiseptic herbal baths will speed up the healing of tears or episiotomies. (See chapter 7, perineal tears; chapter 9, herbal bath.)

Your baby will also be examined to ensure perfect health and this too can be done while still in your arms, if you wish. Although labour is over the third stage is a very important time for you, your husband and your baby. Your baby is at its most alert. You will be, in a sense, meeting each other for the first time, looking into each others eyes and sharing your first hour together.

It is now widely recognised that you need to take your time together, to digest and share your feelings, to celebrate the arrival of a new person to your family, and this bonding is an essential part of your new relationship with each other.

Most of the procedures which need to be done, such as stitching and detailed examination of the baby, can wait for an hour or so.

Try to spend an hour or two together alone (mother, father and baby) immediately after the birth if you are in hospital, and if you are at home this is the appropriate time for the whole family to be together.

'He played on me for an hour and a half, while we talked quietly, my husband and I thoroughly involved in getting to know our new little son. That night we were never separated. He lay calmly looking all around him with a quiet awareness before at last falling asleep. For me those hours will never be forgotten.'

5
Meditation on the Breath

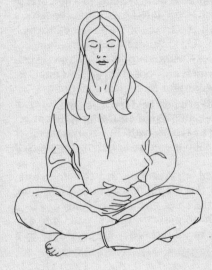

Sitting position for breathing
practice

*'The whole experience was held together for me by a combination
of the upright positions and centring myself with my breathing, and
"tuning in" to my body rhythms. Without this I certainly would not
have had such an enjoyable time.'*

This book does not include any breathing techniques. Our first aim
is to ensure that you are breathing correctly. In the same way that
stiffness is a hidden epidemic in our culture, restricted breathing is
another!

With our civilised way of living our daily life rarely demands that
we use our bodies to their full capacity. Many of us spend our days
without physically exerting ourselves to the extent that our bodies
need in order to stimulate our breathing. The result is that our
breathing becomes shallower and faster than it should normally be,
our supply of oxygen is limited and our elimination of carbon dioxide
is impaired.

If you observe the natural breathing of a baby or a young child you will soon see that the abdomen is moving like a bellows with each breath, while the chest is relatively still and the shoulders are relaxed. This is natural, relaxed deep breathing. By the time we reach adulthood we usually breathe too shallowly using only the upper part of the chest and approximately a third of our capacity of air. By breathing more rapidly than we should we are taking in a new breath before we have emptied our lungs of stale air, so that we have a quantity of stale air mixed with the fresh air we breathe in which decreases our supply of oxygen. This also decreases our vitality.

While we can survive for weeks without solid foods and several days without water, life without air is only possible for a few minutes. Breathing is one of our most important biological functions.

Every living cell absorbs oxygen and expels it in the form of carbon dioxide. If cells of the human brain are completely cut off from fresh oxygen for as little as ten seconds the body can suffer serious harm. In pregnancy and labour you are breathing for yourself and for your baby.

The muscles directly involved in breathing are the intercostal muscles between the ribs and the diaphragm, which is a strong partition of muscle separating the chest and the abdomen.

The lungs themselves contain no muscles, they expand into any empty space with which they are in contact. They are enveloped by a

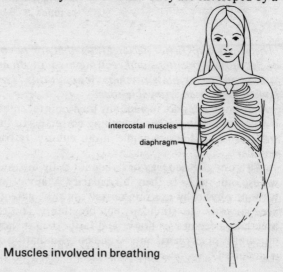

intercostal muscles

diaphragm

Muscles involved in breathing

strong membrane connected with the walls of the chest whose movements cause the lungs to change in volume as air is inhaled and exhaled.

Efficient breathing depends on good posture. If your chest is tight and constricted and your shoulders hunched, the space in your thorax is less and your breathing will be impaired.

Shaped like a vault, the diaphragm muscle flattens out when it works, pressing the abdominal organs downward and arching the abdomen outwards as you breathe in. When you exhale it rests and arches upwards towards the chest cavity.

When we breathe deeply, we use our full thoracic capacity and the diaphragm moves up and down with each breath. This puts mild pressure on the liver, stomach and other internal organs. The rhythm of the lungs is transformed into a gentle massage which promotes the natural functioning of the internal organs. Every breath stimulates the blood circulation to these organs and increases the metabolism. This beneficial massage is lacking when we merely breathe with our upper chest.

So, in fact, we depend upon our breathing for life and health itself – it is the basic rhythm of our bodies. Each time we inhale we are drawing in air – the life-giving element – each time we exhale we are ridding ourselves of waste.

This constant give and take and flow of energy starts the moment we are born and continues throughout our lives, pulsating within us like an alternating current. Every other activity of the body is closely connected with our breathing.

The gateway to the air passages is the nose. Tiny hairs in the nostrils prevent any dust particles from entering the lungs. The nasal passages, lined with mucous membranes, warm the air and filter out dust and germs. Glands fight off bacteria, while our sense of smell protects us from inhaling harmful gases.

Normally we breathe in and out through the nose. In the deep breathing exercise (chapter 2, no. 1) part of the recommended practice is to exhale through the mouth. This is because, during strong contractions in labour, most women naturally tend to breathe out through their mouths. Make a point of breathing in and out through your nose during the day and at night, and breathe out through your mouth only when you practise the deep breathing exercise, or if you feel like it in labour or while stretching.

Regular practice of this exercise will deepen your breathing, helping you to breathe with your whole chest capacity and to use your diaphragm muscle correctly. It will also teach you to concentrate on the basic body rhythm of your breathing. Unlike the rhythm of the heartbeat, or the contractions of the uterus, which take place completely automatically, the rhythm of the breath is the only one which is both voluntary and involuntary. We are able to alter our rate of breathing consciously and this has a direct effect on our state of consciousness.

Your breathing, as you will soon feel, is very closely linked to your mind. In hatha yoga the practice of deep breathing is a prelude to meditation. By turning inwards and focusing your attention on the breath you will have a simple and natural tool for experiencing deeper states of consciousness. This will help you to come into harmony with your inner self and with the deep and intense feelings you will experience in labour. Meditation on the breath stills the mind, stops the internal dialogue that normally spins around our heads, and brings you closer to yourself and your baby inside. Every labour has a rhythm of its own. Concentrating on the rhythm of your breathing will help you to be one with this rhythm, to be instinctive, to surrender to the vital forces working inside your body.

'I was very aware of exactly where the baby was and how my body was doing, and people remarked afterwards how relaxed all my body had been apart from the contracting muscles. Through each contraction I used the deep breathing, at times quite fast and noisily but always with concentration and each time aware of the peak and then the fading of the pain.'

It can be very pleasant and beneficial to you both to practise meditation on the breath together with a partner who will be with you in labour. At first you will feel calmer and more relaxed. Gradually this will deepen to a peaceful meditation which can be very blissful. Women often tell of a deep feeling of ecstasy during a birth. The breath is the key to an awareness of the universal consciousness which is the very essence of life. At a time when one is about to give birth to another being, one is often very much in touch with this divine energy within oneself and all of creation.

'We worship the Holy Breath which is placed higher than all other things created. For lo, the eternal and sovereign luminous space, where rule the unnumbered stars, is the air we breathe in and the air we breathe out. And, in the moment betwixt the breathing in and the breathing out is hidden all the mysteries of the Infinite Garden.'

Jesus Christ, *Essene Gospel of Peace*, Book Two.

6

Massage – The Language of Touch

Combined with movement, position and breathing, massage can be of great use to you in pregnancy and labour. For many people there is nothing as comforting and soothing as the touch of another. Your hands can surprise you with the magic and healing power they contain.

By touching we express our love and affection for each other and we can also effectively use massage to relieve ourselves and others of aches and pains and unnecessary muscle tension.

Massage is an art, which needs to be cultivated, and the only way to learn is through exploration and experiment.

Start on your own body, discover what feels good, which parts of your body need massage and then work with another, preferably someone who will be with you during labour.

There are basically four ways you can touch for massage:

Surface Stroking

This is usually done with the flat of your hand. In severe pain or spasm or in a young baby or child, this very light stroking is often the only form of massage possible.

Deep Stroking

This is done in the same way but more firmly using greater pressure.

Deep Pressure

This is done by pressing firmly with the tips of your fingers or thumbs, even knuckles or elbows, over a small area at a time, getting down deep to tense spots in the body and then using small circular movements to loosen them.

Kneading

This is done by using your whole hand and alternately squeezing and releasing a muscle and is useful over large muscle areas such as buttocks or thighs.

A good starting point is your own hands and feet.

Try This

Explore the skin surface first and then the bony structure underneath. Next explore the range of movement of all the joints, bend your fingers back as far as they can go and then forward. Try feeling each finger and pressing each joint to its limit. Then separate your fingers from side to side. Now explore deeply into the spaces between the bones of the back of your hand and your wrist bones. Lastly shake your hands rapidly, allowing the movement to start from your shoulders, keeping your whole arm loose and relaxed, your wrists completely loose.

Now try your feet in the same way. Try different degrees of pressure, using your thumbs. Press as firmly as you can all the way up the arch of your instep, making small circular movements with your thumb. If you find a painful spot linger on it for a while and try to dissolve the painful sensations. You will probably feel little crystal-like knots of tissue under the skin which yield to the firm massage and seem to disappear. Try the same thing all round the base of your big toe, the sole of your foot and then your heels and Achilles tendon, your ankles and calves. Finally explore the top of your foot and then your toes, one by one, bending them first backwards and then forwards, extending each joint to its limit. Then pull them and twist them and finally separate them from side to side.

Once you have enjoyed massaging your own feet, try treating your partner to a foot massage. You will find that your enjoyment grows and with experience, your own natural inventiveness will lead the way.

Experiment between you with different parts of the body, neck and shoulders, back and front.

Always make sure that you are both completely comfortable.

As your interest grows you will find many good books on massage and courses are also widely available for those who wish to go deeply into the subject.

Massage for Pregnancy

Self Massage

After your bath explore your whole body, perhaps oiling your skin, particularly your belly and breasts, with a good vegetable oil such as almond or wheatgerm. Towards the end of pregnancy it is advisable to oil your perineum with olive oil each day after your bath in preparation for birth.

You will need to know your pelvic area and should frequently explore the bones of your pelvis and massage away any tension in your groin. It is a good idea to be aware of the location of your cervix (try this after bathing, in the squatting position).

While you stretch massage the part of your body where you are feeling the stretch. This is particularly useful for the inner thighs.

Massage by Another

Your partner should start to practise massage for labour while you are pregnant, so that he or she will be able to use massage instinctively to help you during the birth.

To warm up try this.

Head and Neck Massage

Caution
This massage is for pregnancy but the reclining position is not suitable for labour.

Lie down on your back on the floor with your knees bent and legs up on a chair or bed. Place your arms down comfortably by your sides. Your partner sits or kneels behind you making sure that he too is comfortable. (Alternatively you lie down on a bed and he sits on a chair behind you.)

Press downwards on her shoulders with your hands as she breathes out to help her to relax them. Now slip your hands behind her neck and stroke firmly upwards from the base of the neck towards the head, with both hands at once. Lift your hands and repeat a few times, as if lengthening the neck. Go back over the same area but this time make small circles with your fingertips working your way slowly up the neck.

Then lift up her head in your hands and press it slowly and gently upwards and forwards so that her chin comes down towards the breastbone in front of her chest. Hold for a second or two and then slowly lower her head down to the ground. Now turn the head gently to one side and stroke firmly up the side of the neck, end up with firm circular movements at the base of the skull. Linger there for a while then turn the head to the other side and repeat.

Now explore the jaw bone, the upper jaw and mouth, cheeks, cheekbones, nose, temples and the rims of the eye sockets. Make even stroking movements from the centre outwards and then go over the same area making firmer small circular movements and exerting more pressure.

Then stroke the brow from the centre outwards and finally place your hands on either side of the head with your fingers gently covering the eye lids. Sit quietly like this for a minute, both of you breathing deeply and then gently, gently lift your hands.

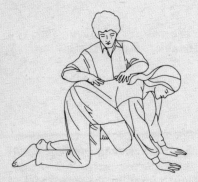

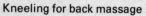
Kneeling for back massage

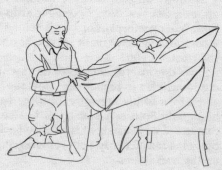

Back Massage

'My husband gently, ever so gently, stroked the lower part of my back and this too was an enormous help.'

Rest comfortably in the kneeling position, leaning forward onto a pile of cushions, with your knees apart and your feet pointing towards each other. Your partner should kneel down behind you keeping his or her own back straight.

Alternatively sit facing backwards on a chair, your partner can kneel behind you on the floor or sit on a chair.

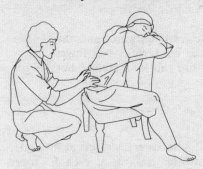

Sitting backwards on a chair for
back massage

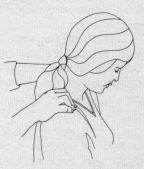

Kneading the shoulder
muscles

Start at the base of the skull and feel each vertebra of the spine massaging each one in small circles until you reach the sacrum. Then using the thumbs of each hand, massage the muscles on the sides of the spinal column using as firm a pressure as your partner can enjoy, again make small circular movements. Linger on the tense spots.

Then place your hands on the soft muscles in the shoulders and knead until tension yields.

During labour the lower back in the sacral area is the part that most needs massage. It is best to massage during a contraction and then to stop in between. Use a pleasant talcum powder to avoid stickiness. Most women do not enjoy deep pressure massage during contractions but prefer a light stroking. Try to use slow rhythmic strokes which harmonise with her breathing. The best way to practise this is to breathe deeply yourself while you massage. Using the flat surface of your palm, particularly the heel, make light, slow, rhythmic circles over the sacral area.

'*When I was in transition I became a bit panicky and here I found my husband Brian very helpful because he reminded me to keep taking deep, slow breaths. All through the contractions he gently and lightly massaged my lower back and this I found a marvellous distraction from the pain.*'

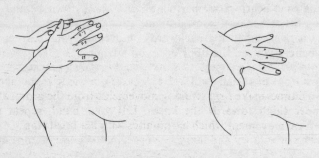

Circular massage for lower back

Now try using the palms of both hands and starting at the centre make slow even movements outwards towards or even down her thighs. Then lift your hands and repeat.

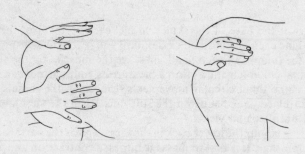

Side stroking for the lower back

Now try to cup one hand over the lower end of the spine so that the heel of your palm covers her coccyx. Keeping your hand still, exert slight pressure so that the warmth of your hand spreads into her back. Some women find this helpful during contractions.

'The heat from Ron's hand just laid on the base of my spine was so soothing and he could feel the coccyx lift.'

Place the palm of your left hand at the top of the spine and make a firm stroking movement down to the sacrum. Then do the same with your right hand and repeat rhythmically alternating hands. This is very calming and can be used to quieten the shivers and may also be useful during bearing down.

Thigh, Calf and Foot Massage

Sit comfortably, leaning forward slightly. Your partner should kneel in front of you in a comfortable position. Using both hands at the same time, make firm stroking movements from the groin, along the inner thigh towards the knees. Lift your hand, repeat in a rhythmical movement which harmonises with her breathing.

During pregnancy and labour, you may experience cramps in the calf muscles. Sitting on a chair place one foot in your partner's lap. Your partner should bend your foot/toes up towards your leg, take hold of the calf muscle and gently knead with his hand.

Now pass on to the foot. This can also be done in the kneeling position. During labour foot massage can be extremely helpful, particularly in the area of the heel and the Achilles tendon.

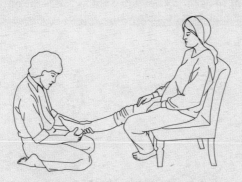

Massage for heel and Achilles tendon

Take the foot in one hand and, using the other hand, make smooth circles over both sides of the heel, and then even strokes on either side of the Achilles tendon. Explore the ankle bone and use deep pressure here to find tender spots. For some people deep massage at the base of the ankle bone can help to lessen labour pains if you find the right spot.

Belly Massage

During labour, while you are experiencing the intense sensations of a contraction, you may find a light fingertip massage over your lower abdomen soothing. Try this yourself in the standing position.

In a half circle, make a very gentle sweeping movement over your lower belly from one side to the other. Lift your hand and repeat in harmony with your breathing.

Now try this with a partner.

Lastly, your partner should become familiar with the parts of your body which generally tense up when you are under stress and be able instinctively to stroke away tension in labour, be it a frown on your forehead, tense raised shoulders, clenched fists or whatever.

Most women enjoy the relaxing effect of massage in labour. However, you may find that you prefer not to be touched when the time comes.

You might prefer a very light touch, or you might enjoy a deeper pressure. Make your likes and dislikes known to your partner and don't be afraid to ask for what you want as this is the only way he or she will know how best to help you.

7

Active Birth at Home or in Hospital

Choosing the Place of Birth

There is no way of removing every risk in childbirth. Although the vast majority of babies are born safely, the final outcome of any birth is always uncertain. Unexpected complications can arise, machines can break down, anyone can make a mistake. There is no evidence to prove that either home or hospital is safer. However, different factors such as your health, age, whether you have any problems in pregnancy and what choices are available to you, will help to determine the best place of birth for you.

The important thing is to discover all the possibilities, to consider what your priorities are, then to make a choice which feels right for you. Your instinctive feelings are really important – think of a cat and how she will find just the right corner to have her kittens! The choices are:

a. A home birth.
b. A GP unit where you have your baby in hospital but under the care of your own GP with your local community midwives attending you. The hospital would take over only in the event of complications arising and you can go back home after six hours with your baby if all is well. Many women find this a good way to give birth actively in hospital and enjoy the more homely atmosphere and the familiarity of a doctor and midwife whom they know well. This system has proved so satisfactory that the Health Service plans to expand the availability of this choice in the next two years.
c. Then there is the choice of a consultant hospital. (Some of these have some GP beds too.)

If you would like more information and advice on the choices available see chapter 9 for some useful addresses and contacts. If you have any of the following problems you may need to have your baby in hospital:

Toxaemia or pre-eclampsia
This occurs when blood pressure rises to dangerous levels. It does not mean a slight rise in blood pressure which is quite common at the end of pregnancy and needs careful observation but generally presents no problems unless it continues to rise or rises sharply. Blood pressure is connected with the emotions and sometimes the excitement of approaching the birth can cause a slight rise. (See chapter 9 for prevention and treatment of high blood pressure.)

Breech presentation
There are more risks involved than in a normal presentation. (See Unusual Presentations under Active Birth in Hospital.)

Previous complications
Not all complications are likely to recur. However, if there were problems with the last birth which could affect this one then you are better off in hospital.

Placenta praevia
Sometimes the placenta lies in the lower abdomen and is actually close to or covering the cervix. Here the danger is that the placenta could separate and be born before the baby and result in the baby being cut off from its source of nourishment.

Although a low-lying placenta often ends in a perfectly normal birth, it is necessary to have help close at hand in case a Caesarean is required. (With a real placenta praevia a Caesarean is always necessary.)

Active Birth at Home

'There was a feeling of great calm and peace and relaxation around and we all lay down together in our family bed for the night. It felt so good not to have any separation either from Kurt or David.'

There are many advantages to a home birth. In your own home you are the centre around which everything else revolves, rather than a patient, dependent on the routines of a large institution. Your attendants come into your home as guests. You can relax in the comfort and security of a familiar atmosphere with your loved ones around you. The birth is an event in your family life, a special occasion, a time to celebrate. For the other children in the family, particularly if they are very young, a home birth is of great value as they can welcome their new brother or sister without the pain of a separation from you. Some families choose to have their children present at the actual birth and in this way completely included in the experience.

'As he was born and we were waiting for the cord to stop pulsating I suddenly became more aware of how wonderful it was, for us all to be together at this time – the girls at 9 and 10 years had witnessed the birth of their brother in a very bonding experience.'

In pregnancy you have the great advantage of continuity of care. There is plenty of time to get to know the midwife or midwives who are going to attend you and to discuss your wishes with them in advance. You can also have the comfort of your own family doctor present at the birth. Make the most of the many opportunities to discuss what you intend to do with your doctor or midwife. It will help you enormously to approach the birth with confidence if you feel that you can trust your attendants to support and encourage you to give birth actively. If this is their first experience of active birth then lend them this book!

'The prospect of even small difficulty ahead suddenly daunted me and being at home in loving arms made it easier for me to protest that I couldn't face it. In hospital, in being geared to fight off interference, I was also fully geared to fight my own weakness, whereas at home it was safer for me to want to give up.'

If you are hoping for a natural birth you can avoid routine hospital practices and there is less temptation at home to resort to drugs or intervention in your weaker moments. You are the only person in labour, the birth process can unfold naturally, you can take your time and are not subjected to the inconvenience of moving to hospital. You can create the ideal environment for yourself, use the bathroom whenever you want to, make as much noise as you want to, listen to music or not and help yourself to food or drink of your choice. It is possible to have complete bodily freedom and to give birth either in your own bed or on the floor. You can be alone or share the experience with people of your own choosing. After the birth you can all be together to enjoy the special time of celebration in the family.

You can sleep when your baby sleeps and have your baby with you in bed day or night. It is usually easier to establish breastfeeding and to learn to care for your baby in these conditions.

Medically speaking you are expected to fall into the 'low risk' category and should be in good health with no problems in your pregnancy and no history of illness or obstetric complications which could affect the birth.

Arrange a suitable back-up in advance in case complications arise and you need to be transferred to hospital.

The birth room

'I went upstairs to the bedroom which I had prepared for the birth. There was a foam mattress in front of the fire, covered with a clean sheet, an enormous beanbag also covered with a sheet resting against the foot of my bed and a small stool to sit on between contractions.'

Arrange a pleasant environment where you have several alternatives for changing positions. There is no special equipment needed – most homes will have everything you need already. Make sure you have a good supply of cushions and a low stool or pile of books for squatting on.

The room should be warm with extra heating available for the actual birth as the baby will need to be kept very warm after birth.

The lighting should be comfortable. Dim light is most conducive for relaxation in labour with one lamp or angle-poise light handy for the midwife in case she needs it. Your midwife or local clinic will provide you with a maternity box for the delivery. (Useful for the supply of cotton wool alone.)

Make full use of the bath tub or shower. It is unlikely that your baby will be born in the water, however, it is perfectly all right if it does happen.

'I decided to relax in a bath. On feeling a contraction I stepped out of it to lean against the sink and to slowly rotate my body as if twisting a hoola-hoop. I continued in this way topping-up the bath with hot water until I had three consecutive contractions each lasting about a minute.'

A portable sonicaid heart monitor, if your GP has one, will increase the safety factor.

Have a baby bath or a large plastic tub ready in the bathroom in case you decide to bath the baby immediately after birth. Also have a large jug or bucket handy as the temperature of the water may need adjusting. The water should be warm as the baby has been used to your body temperature, but not too hot.

After the birth it is not necessary to dress the baby until the next day. Have plenty of soft wrapping blankets handy – soft flannel sheets would be fine – as the baby needs to be kept warm. For the first day or two after the birth (or longer) it is best for the baby to be close to the familiar sound of your heartbeat. It is perfectly safe for you to sleep together and to bath together at this time.

In the hours after the birth your midwife will help to clear up and then she will leave. It's worth thinking in advance of what you will need at that time and have it all handy at your bedside beforehand. Mainly you will need a bowl for warm water and cotton wool to clean the baby when the first bowel movement occurs. This is usually dark green, or a black sticky substance called meconium. In a day or so the bowel movement will become a yellowish colour. You will need nappies of some sort. Disposables in the tiniest size are handy and save you having to wash nappies at first. You need plenty of them! It is also a good idea to have some almond oil to put on your nipples after the baby sucks. This will help prevent soreness. (See chapter 9, Breasts & Breastfeeding.)

You will probably be feeling marvellous after the birth, but take care to be getting enough rest and sleep and to use your energy for your baby. Without the protection of hospital visiting hours one can find oneself entertaining visitors all day after a home birth. You need plenty of time to get to know your new baby quietly in the days after the birth.

If you have difficulty in arranging a home birth then see chapter 9 for some useful addresses and contacts who may be able to help.

Active Birth in Hospital

There is no reason why active birth cannot be put into practice in any environment suitable for a birth. Indeed there are several hospitals in London and elsewhere in the country where women who have prepared for active birth have managed successfully to give birth in this way. If you are having your baby in hospital, do find out beforehand whether they will allow you to move around and use natural positions for delivery. It is advisable for you and your partner to make an appointment to see the consultant under whom you are booked and then have your wishes written on your card with his or her consent. Do ask questions about everything you want to know as many hospitals will be willing to accommodate you. It is wise to talk to the senior nursing officer who is head of midwifery as she will be most familiar with the way the labour ward is run.

More hospitals are recognising the advantages of active birth although there are many which still deny women the right to choose a natural birth. In various hospitals some of the staff support this right and others do not. It is important for you to find out the situation well in advance and it is your right to change to a hospital which suits your needs. As already mentioned the GP unit system is often the best way to have an active birth in hospital, and has the great advantage of continuity of care and gives you an early opportunity to discuss your wishes with the midwives and your doctor.

'I had previously stated that I wanted no enema, monitor, drugs or cuts unless absolutely necessary and once the midwife had confirmed my wishes, no more was said.'

Whether you are having your baby at home or in hospital you will need good antenatal care and education during your pregnancy.

What to take with you

Take a large, firm floor cushion or two (measuring roughly three feet square) with you to lean on, as the small pillows usually provided by the hospital do not offer enough support. The cushion should be firm and as high as possible and, of course, very clean. You will need several hospital pillows as well. Ask for extra pillows when you arrive.

Most hospital delivery rooms have a stool which is used for getting up onto the bed. This is perfect for squatting. Place one of the pillows on it or ask the midwife for a sterile paper pad. The delivery table, although not ideal, is usually quite narrow, but is wide enough to kneel or squat on reasonably comfortably. The bars at the back of the delivery table come in very handy for holding onto while kneeling or squatting, and if the whole bed is pulled forward by a few inches your partner can also stand behind the bed to support you.

Most delivery beds are adjustable – they can usually be lowered, the back can be raised and sometimes the end and the backrest can be removed altogether. Explore these possibilities in advance. (We keep hearing from people of new ways in which they have managed to use whatever is available at the time.) If the staff will allow, your partner can sit on the bed with you in order to support or massage you.

Although the delivery bed is rather high, and will restrict your movement to some extent, which is not ideal, it does allow you to be easily supported and your attendants can reach and see very easily. Some hospitals in London prefer to place a mattress on the floor for women who wish to squat or have a squatting birth stool. This is very helpful.

Make a tour of the labour ward beforehand, notice the whereabouts of bathrooms and showers so you can make use of them during your labour. It is also a good idea to take a pad for kneeling on. A piece of foam rubber two inches thick in a clean pillow case is ideal. Then you can kneel on the floor or use it on the bed to protect your knees.

Many couples like to take a tape recorder with music of their choice, and this is often quite delightfully relaxing for the attendants as well.

Take your own nightgown to wear as you will want to look and feel good. A short cotton one which can open in front is ideal and easy to take off. You will need a sponge (natural if possible) and a face cloth for wiping your face in between contractions, and a fan in hot weather. If the room is overheated (often the case in hospital) try turning down the radiators.

You may like to take your own tea bags for herbal tea (camomile or raspberry leaf) and a jar of pure honey. A spoonful every now and then in herbal tea will ensure that your blood sugar level doesn't drop, and eliminate the need for a glucose drip. Natural apple juice or red grape juice will have the same effect, as will glucose tablets (don't take citrus juice – it's too acidic). Of course, your partner will need some food and some coins for the call box.

Movements for labour

You will probably be advised to stay at home for the first part of the first stage and hopefully you will arrive in hospital to find yourself already dilating. When you arrive you will be admitted, examined and offered an enema, a shave and a bath. It is possible to refuse the enema and shave if you would rather not have them, as they are not necessary. Shaving, besides being quite humiliating for some women, often causes infections when the growing hairs irritate the healing tissues of the perineum after birth.

A bath or shower is very relaxing – don't rush, enjoy it! Many labour wards have showers and if you have a long first stage you may enjoy making use of them from time to time. You can walk around the delivery room or up and down the corridor. When labour gets stronger you may like to stand at the side of the delivery bed, place your big cushion in front of you and lean forward onto it for contractions, using the stool for one foot. Another good idea is to sit on a chair facing the bed and lean forward onto it.

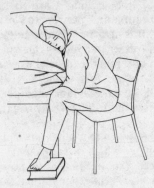

Sitting position for labour

You can use the stool for squatting, or squat on the floor holding onto the bar of the bed for support. When labour gets very strong you can get up on the delivery bed if you are expected or want to do so. Lift up the backrest and pile your cushions up against it so that you can lean forward onto the cushions and rest completely supported in the kneeling position between contractions.

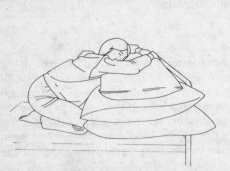

Kneeling forward onto cushions

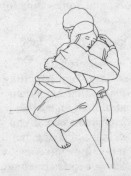

Supported squatting on the delivery bed

You can squat holding on to the backrest. Alternatively, your partner can stand behind the bed to support you – or at the side. Try squatting sideways on the bed putting your arms around your partner's shoulders for support.

You could also face the other way and squat leaning forward. Follow your instincts to adapt the environment to suit your needs. It is a good idea to practise on the kitchen table beforehand!

The second stage in hospital

The kneeling position presents no problem on a bed, simply kneel forward onto a pile of cushions. If you are able to remain on the floor you can follow the advice given in chapter 4 for the second stage. At the time of writing this book many hospitals insist that the second stage take place on a bed. If this is the case for you these are the ways of being supported in a squatting position on a bed.

Squatting with two people supporting

'Very soon after arrival I felt like pushing, was examined and found to be fully dilated. Contractions were now coming almost continuously and I squatted throughout, supported by my husband and an extra doctor who had come along to watch.'

Squat on the bed. Place a pillow under your heels as this will make squatting easier. Your supporters should stand at your sides on either side of the bed. If they are more or less the same height you will probably be able to put one arm round each of their shoulders quite comfortably. They can each put one arm round your back and use the other arm to support you under each knee, if this is comfortable for you.

For variation and resting you can come forward into a kneeling position. It is also possible to stand up during contractions by holding on to your supporters' shoulders.

'I was helped by the doctor and my husband into a squatting position. This was marvellous! I could push so much easier and it was a comfort to feel their strength helping support me. I stayed squatting as this brought her head down very quickly.'

If the midwife is not used to this position and wants to see the perineum more clearly, then your supporters can move back a little to allow you to lean back a bit.

In some hospitals, at the time of writing, midwives were prepared to allow squatting up until the crowning of the baby's head but not for

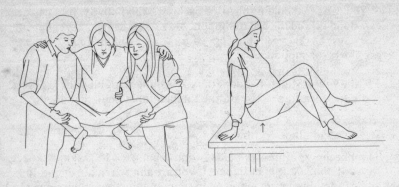

Supported squatting on the bed   Compromise position

the actual delivery. In this case, sit upright when the crowning begins, with your hands behind you and your feet down in front of you. If you can, lift yourself up a little with your hands as the baby comes out. In this position your body is upright, your weight is on your buttock bones rather than your sacrum and you can use your arms and legs to help you. Many hospitals will agree to this compromise. If not try the side-lying position rather than the semi-reclining.

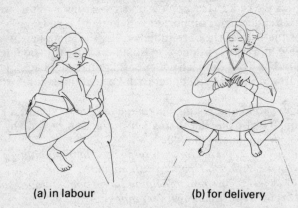

(a) in labour   (b) for delivery

Supported squat from behind the bed

Another way to support you in the squatting position is from behind. This has worked well in a situation where it was possible to lower the backrest. Your partner can stand behind the bed and support you as in the 'standing squat' in chapter 4.

This can also be done (and is possibly more comfortable) if the mother squats sideways on the bed, if the midwife is willing to assist from the other side.

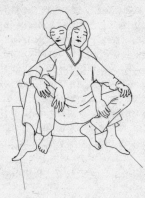

Supported squatting with the partner seated on cushions on the bed

Another possibility is if the supporter sits on the pile of cushions on the bed behind the mother. Then she can squat between his legs using his body for support.

These examples are all drawn from situations where people have managed to find their own ways of making use of whatever is available and acceptable to the hospital. It is important to visit the labour room beforehand to get an idea of the possibilities and to discuss them with the staff.

Monitoring the Baby for Active Birth

This means checking your baby's heartbeat and needs to be done regularly during pregnancy and labour. It is possible to hear the baby's heartbeat clearly by placing one's ear against the abdomen. The ordinary ear trumpet is perfectly adequate and the midwife may ask you to sit up vertically or lean back slightly while she uses it. Some enterprising midwives manage to use it from underneath while the woman in labour kneels. The stethoscope is perhaps easier to use in this position. The best type of monitor is the doptone, or sonicaid heart monitor. These are relatively inexpensive and most hospitals have one. They can be used with the woman in any upright position and cause no discomfort to mother or baby. There is no evidence that the ultra-sound waves used affect the baby but it is still under-researched. There are portable doptone monitors which can be used at home. You hear the sound of the baby's heartbeat magnified which can be very reassuring.

The abdominal belt monitors most commonly used at the time of writing present certain problems. They involve the mother wearing two belts strapped around her abdomen – one to measure the contractions, and one the baby's heartbeat – which generally confines her to the semi-reclining position. Many women complain that these are very uncomfortable. The contractions are more painful and also there is a real contradiction here – the monitors are meant to detect any foetal distress while confining the mother to the position most likely to induce it! Also we know that machines often break down and don't work properly, and when midwives rely solely on machinery their instincts to detect distress suffer.

Women from our classes have successfully used belt monitors in the kneeling position which helps to solve some of the problems.

'I had to get onto the delivery bed and be monitored, as the doctor was worried as the baby was small. As soon as I lay down on the bed the contractions were painful and so as soon as the monitors were attached I turned over and knelt up on the bed facing the wall. Immediately the pain disappeared and I could cope well with the contractions.'

The other form of monitoring very commonly used, often in addition to the belt monitor, is the scalp electrode. These are attached by a tiny screw or hook to the baby's scalp through the cervix. This form of monitoring allows the mother greater mobility depending on the length of the flex and the flexibility of the attendants. However, the disadvantage here is that the membranes have to be artificially ruptured in order to attach the monitor, and this has its attendant risks – it will accelerate labour, sometimes violently. Rupturing the membranes also causes unnecessary pressure from the contracting uterus on the infant's head (see chapter 9, Artificial Rupture of Membranes). Their comfort for the baby, as a first touch from the outside world, is also questionable. Some babies are left with a small wound and occasionally a permanent tiny bald patch where the electrode was attached. In the event of a real complication (such as the baby being distressed) though, it is important to weigh up these problems against the risks of not using them and work out one's priorities.

There is a new form of radio operated monitoring (telemetry) currently being marketed which allows complete mobility but still necessitates rupturing the membranes to attach a scalp electrode.

It is essential that the system of monitoring should not disrupt the normal physiology of labour. As soon as this is the case the monitor itself can become the cause of the problems it is intended to prevent.

Internal Examinations

These are done by the midwife to assess the progress of the labour. She will insert her hand into your vagina and feel the cervix and the top of the baby's head to gather information about the dilation and the presentation of the baby.

When birth is active and labour is obviously progressing well it is not necessary to make these examinations often, and sometimes not at all. Most midwives like to examine internally at the end of the first stage to check if dilation is complete. You may wish to be examined to know how far you have dilated yourself.

Some women do not mind being examined but others often complain that it is uncomfortable to be touched in this most tender part during labour. Internal examinations can be done very gently between, rather than during, contractions and in a position most comfortable to you. It is possible to examine a woman standing up (with one leg up on a chair), sitting on the edge of a chair or kneeling forward on all fours.

'The hospital staff agreed to and managed examinations with me sitting on the edge of a chair. And regularly the baby's heartbeat was checked with a portable monitor – which hardly interrupted me at all.'

This will be far less uncomfortable than turning over into the semi-reclining position.

Usually midwives have been trained to examine in a semi-reclining position and often do not like to change their ways, which is understandable in such a responsible job. Perhaps you could ask her to try another position first, agreeing to turn over if she has any difficulty and then she will probably discover that it is just as good.

If, for some reason, she requires you to turn round, it cannot harm you to do so (the movement could probably help you) and you can turn back again when she has finished. Breathing deeply and relaxing as much as possible while being examined should help.

The kneeling position offers attendants an excellent view of what is happening as the baby is born. In fact, as far as view and access go this position is ideal. The problem here is that the midwife's routine is literally turned upside down – but there should be little difficulty. When dealing with spontaneous birth in which the woman follows her own instincts, the midwifery is also by necessity more spontaneous and more instinctive. In the few places in the western world where birth is managed this way the statistics are so much better than those of our high technology hospitals that there is justification for the argument that spontaneous midwifery is safest and best and more satisfying for all concerned.

In the squatting position the midwife will need to rely on her hands to feel the baby's progress, or else bend down to look. As the pelvis is more open and the perineum more relaxed in this position there is less need for examination and rarely any need to guard the perineum.

After the baby's head emerges the midwife will check with her finger to see if the umbilical cord is round the baby's neck. It is a common occurrence and all the midwife will normally have to do is to loosen the cord by pulling it a little and slip it over the baby's head as it emerges, or just after. Midwives with experience of the squatting position tell us that this presents no problems and can be handled in exactly the same way as if the mother was reclining.

In the rare case of the cord being wound twice or more times around the neck it is safest for the mother to be squatting in this instance (preferably a standing squat), as the pelvis will be wide open and the baby will be born much quicker than if the mother were reclining. Cutting the cord is not desirable in this situation, unless it is preventing the baby from coming out, and in this circumstance the squatting or kneeling position is imperative. Normally, once the child is born the cord is quickly unravelled and left to stop pulsating while the baby is passed to its mother.

Accelerating Labour

If labour is very slow there is usually no cause for concern provided the baby's heartbeat is normal, the mother is coping and feeling well, and the labour is progressing. Many women need to take a long time sinking into the first stage, and others need time to let the baby descend to be born in the second stage. In a slow labour immersion in water is often very helpful. Walking, perhaps outdoors if the weather permits, can help.

As far as movement and posture goes, the more vertical postures will help the baby to descend and exert more pressure on the cervix. Squatting is most likely to intensify the contractions. Movement will probably accelerate the labour and half kneeling half squatting can speed up dilation of the cervix. It often happens that progress is very slow and suddenly advances rapidly – it could be 12 hours going from 0–6 cm and 10 minutes from 6 cm to full dilation. Sometimes hunger can cause delay. Perhaps the mother is afraid of something she cannot express, or is struggling inwardly with unconscious inhibitions. If she is given understanding and space she will probably find her own way of overcoming her difficulties.

It is quite normal for some labours to stop and start during the first stage. If labour is not progressing after a long time has elapsed, and there does not seem to be an obvious reason, one should allow for the possibility that there may be some physical problem such as the presentation of the baby or the internal shape of the mother's pelvis, and help may be needed.

Slowing Down Labour

If labour is progressing very fast then the kneeling position on hands and knees can help the woman to stay in control. The knee-chest position may help to slow down the contractions. Very slow deep breathing will be helpful.

Unusual Presentations

Usually before birth the baby lies with its head engaged in the pelvis in what is known as the anterior position. The baby's back will be lying against your abdominal wall and the limbs will be folded in front facing your spine. The head will be flexed well forward ready for birth. In this position the baby's descent through the birth canal will be easiest. However, sometimes there are variations in the way the baby lies which can cause difficulty during labour and birth.

With the use of natural upright positions these variations can usually be managed without intervention. When the mother is moving in labour there is more likelihood of the baby being able to move into the correct position.

Posterior presentation

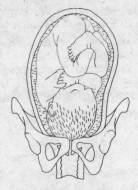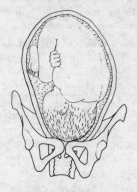

Drawing of baby in
posterior position

Drawing of baby in
anterior position

In the posterior position the baby is lying with its spine against your spine and its limbs facing towards your abdominal wall. Often the baby will rotate into the anterior position when labour begins but sometimes remains posterior for the birth. With the use of natural positions this doesn't usually present any serious problems, however, there is more pressure from the baby's head on the mother's sacrum which usually results in a 'backache labour'. The fit between the baby's head and the pelvis isn't quite as perfect so the labour can be somewhat slower. The instinctive way to deal with a posterior presentation is to kneel forward so that the weight of the baby is taken off the mother's back which eases the pain. Rotating the hips will help the baby to descend. Standing up, leaning forward and rotating the hips is also useful.

For the second stage squatting or a standing squat are best, allowing maximum opening of the pelvis and help from gravity. Sometimes the kneeling position is most comfortable and practical for the delivery.

Breech presentation

When a baby is lying in a breech position its head is uppermost and its bottom or legs are presenting first.

It is quite possible for a baby to be born in this position but there

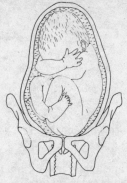

Breech presentation

are ways of gently encouraging a breech baby to turn before labour starts. It is desirable to do so as a breech birth is problematic in that the head of the baby is the largest part of its body and will be emerging last. If there is any delay this can be dangerous.

If you discover that your baby is breech by the fourth week before labour is due, stop squatting and try this exercise. (Discuss this with your doctor or midwife before you start to be sure that it is safe for you.) A word of caution; lots of babies are lying breech 6 weeks before and then turn spontaneously, so don't do anything until 4 weeks beforehand.

Caution
If you find that you are dizzy lying on your back then you should not do these exercises – try to spend time in the knee-chest position instead (see chapter 4, page 82).

Exercises to encourage a breech baby to turn
It is important not to use force but to attempt certain movements oneself which may gently persuade your baby to turn. If the baby insists on remaining in the breech position then allow nature to take its course. First of all discuss this exercise with your doctor or midwife and ask them to help you to feel how your baby is lying before you start. Discover the exact location of the head, the limbs, the baby's spine and the placenta, if you can.

1. Place a large firm cushion or two on the floor and lie down on your back with your hips raised up on the cushion and your head on the floor so that your pelvis is higher than your head. You can place a pillow under your head.

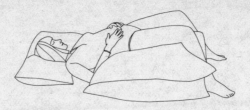

Drawing of exercise to turn a breech (No. 1)

In this position the baby will drop slightly away from the pelvis and may begin to move. Lie like this for ten minutes several times throughout the day. Relax and breathe deeply. Massage your belly with your hands and try gently to encourage your baby to turn. In many ways this is a matter of communication between you and your baby, and usually takes a week or two before the baby turns. When it happens you will probably feel that there is a change. Arrange beforehand with your doctor or midwife that as soon as you suspect that the baby has turned you can have an examination. If this confirms that the head is down then stop doing the exercise and start squatting in order to help the head to engage.

2. If the baby's bottom is actually engaged in the pelvic brim then what is needed is simply to get your bottom up higher than your head in order to disengage the baby. You need someone to assist you and, ideally, your midwife to help. This is the best position to disengage a breech. (It works on the simple principle that if something is stuck in a hole, turn it upside down to loosen it.) You need a chair and a cushion on the chair. Lie on your back on the floor. Bend your knees, take hold of the front legs of the chair with your hands and perhaps with the help of someone strong, lift up your hips onto the chair adjusting the cushion to make yourself comfortable.

Try this exercise only once or twice, do not repeat it frequently. In this position the baby will drop down out of the pelvis. You can massage gently with your hands to help the baby to disengage by stroking from your pubic bone upwards towards your navel. Soon you will feel that your lower abdomen is empty. Gently remove the chair and place a large cushion under your hips and carry on with exercise 1.

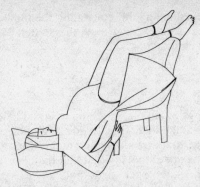

Drawing of exercise to disengage a breech (No. 2)

Usually after this a baby will turn. However, if your baby is still breech in labour then, if your obstetrician is agreeable, stay vertical and squat fully to bear down in order to give your baby as much room as possible and to get maximum help from gravity.

Michel Odent stresses that in the case of a breech the supported standing squat is imperative for delivery. The problem with a breech is that the head of the baby is the largest part and as this is coming last any delay could be dangerous. The standing squat allows for rapid descent of the baby through the pelvis. Odent believes that this method of delivering a breech is safer than a forceps delivery where there is always a risk of damage to the baby from the forceps.

Transverse presentation

If your baby is lying transverse by the fourth week before labour is due, then do the same exercise (1.) as for breech. Kneeling and rotating your hips for the first stage may help to get your baby into the correct position. If this happens then squat if you can for the second stage.

There are a few very rare instances where the baby's head is at an unusual angle with the neck extended rather than flexed. This can lead to a situation where the head cannot pass through your pelvis, however, this is less likely to happen if you are moving your own body intuitively during labour.

It is most important to have a thorough pelvic examination in early pregnancy as it is helpful to know that the shape and size of your pelvis does not present any difficulty. This is supposed to be part of the routine check in early pregnancy but is often overlooked in the busier antenatal clinics.

Perineal Tears

In the second stage of labour, as the baby's head comes down to the base of the pelvis and crowns, the perineal tissues between the vagina and anus fan out and stretch open. In the squatting or kneeling position the pelvis opens to its widest and the back or sacral part of the pelvic floor draws backwards and is in a passive state of relaxation, allowing maximum opening of the vagina. In this position a tear is less likely than if you are reclining. However, tears are a natural hazard of birth. They usually heal without difficulty but the stitching to repair them can be uncomfortable and sometimes painful.

How to avoid a tear

- During pregnancy practise stretching exercises and pelvic floor exercises regularly.
- In the last six weeks massage the perineum and the whole vaginal area with olive oil after your bath. Some midwives recommend stretching the perineum with your fingers.
- Use upright squatting or kneeling positions for the birth of the baby.
- Don't rush or push forcefully in the second stage. Let your uterus be your guide and follow your own urges to deliver your child. If you don't try to hurry the process your perineum will generally have time to fan out and relax.
- Ask the midwife not to swab you down with disinfectant as this simply washes away the natural lubrication and will make a tear more likely.
- In natural positions it is generally not necessary for the midwife to guard the perineum. However, if the tissues seem very tight it is very helpful to apply hot towels. A small towel (a good way to break in the new nappies) can be used. Take several and pour boiling water over them in a basin. As soon as they are touchable, wring them out, fold and place over the perineum. This is very soothing and will help to bring blood to the area and relax the

tissues. Possibly the 'all fours' kneeling position would be best for this as the perineum is uppermost.

● Use your own hands to feel the baby's head when it begins to crown and to ease the tissues or even massage them with a little oil. Interestingly, mothers who use their own hands to help the baby out rarely tear!

Repairing a tear

Sometimes a small tear will not need stitching. If it does, however, it is definitely advisable, though, to have a local anaesthetic to deaden the pain as this is not going to affect your baby. Make sure you don't feel anything and ask for more anaesthetic if you do – even one stitch can be very painful without an injection. Also, ensure that whoever is doing the stitching has plenty of experience and can do a good job. (See chapter 9 for a marvellous herbal remedy to soothe and promote healing in the days to come.)

It is not necessary to have your legs up in stirrups while a tear is being repaired and, in fact, you can probably relax better with your legs apart and knees bent.

Episiotomy

An episiotomy is a surgical incision or cut which is made in the perineum with scissors to enlarge the vaginal opening. A local anaesthetic is injected into the area beforehand so that the incision is painless. The cut is roughly ½–1 inch long and is made through skin and muscle of the perineum, either down the midline or at an angle, and is sewn up after the birth (whereas a natural tear is more superficial and does not go through the muscle layer).

The need to intervene in this way is certainly the exception rather than the rule but with the advance of modern ostetrics episiotomy has become a routine procedure which is now done in this country to almost 100 per cent of all first-time mothers, and between 30–70 per cent of all deliveries.

In 1981 the National Childbirth Trust published a booklet on episiotomy edited by Sheila Kitzinger which is essential reading for any mother-to-be and her attendants (see chapter 9, Recommended Reading). The results of their survey show that generally episiotomy is unnecessary and that a natual tear heals better and presents less physical and psychological problems than a cut. In our work we have exactly the same findings.

When birth is active and natural upright positions are used for the second stage, when the mother is encouraged to take her time and follow her own instincts, rather than to push forcefully, the need for an episiotomy is greatly reduced. It is only in rare situations where the perineum is especially tight, or if an episiotomy will be life-saving for the baby by speeding up the delivery that it is really necessary. When birth is active episiotomy takes its rightful place as an emergency procedure.

In combination with active birth in such a situation, the 'all fours' kneeling position is the best posture to use when an episiotomy is required. In this way the baby is receiving a better supply of oxygen as there is no pressure on the internal blood vessels. The mother is more comfortable. The perineal tissues are most accessible and relaxed, and there is less danger of extended tearing after the cut is made as there is less pressure on the perineum as the baby's head emerges. If the baby is distressed the greater opening of the pelvic outlet in this position would help to speed up the delivery. It is important if you have an episiotomy that the stitching be done soon after the birth to prevent blood loss, infection and to promote healing. Local anaesthetic is essential.

Many professionals now recognise that episiotomies are performed unnecessarily, however, the routine use of this operation is still widespread. It is the most common of all obstetric operations and is often done without the consent of a healthy woman who may not need it at all. As the after-effects can be very painful and the actual operation, though brief, can disturb and interrupt one of the most intimate and deeply personal experiences of your life, it is well worth discussing this subject with your attendants before the event and having your wishes written on your medical card.

'We obstetricians teach that episiotomy prevents tears and reduces the likelihood of prolapse in the future – but we have little or no evidence for making these statements. Not only is there no evidence that episiotomy prevents tears but there is some evidence to the contrary ...'

M. J. House, MRCOG, consultant obstetrician,
from *Episiotomy – Physical and Emotional Aspects*,
National Childbirth Trust, 1981.

Active Birth and Obstetrics

It has often happened that women have managed successfully to combine active birth with obstetric help. The following are some examples.

Induction

With active birth the need to induce labour artificially is reduced. However, if you have symptoms of pre-eclampsia or if your baby must be born without delay – that is, if induction is medically indicated – then prostoglandin suppositories or oral syntocinon are best for active labour as they will not restrict your movement. Normally, once labour is induced careful monitoring is necessary.

A drip can be applied in the kneeling position and this will be very helpful to you in coping with the contractions which are often far more intense and violent than the natural ones. Some hospitals have mobile drips which enable you to walk or stand up. The heart monitor can also be worn in this position. (See also chapter 9, Induction.)

'Although my son's birth was induced I found plenty of opportunity to use the all-fours position, using a rocking motion during contractions and resting back on my heels with knees well apart, and meditating in between.'

Epidurals

Side lying is preferable to semi-reclining, but change sides frequently. You can sit upright and lean forward slightly or sit on the edge of the bed and lean forward with the midwife's assistance. Changing positions is extremely beneficial as epidurals often cause loss of muscle power and therefore less efficient contractions. For delivery, side lying is preferable to lying back or, if the epidural has worn off, you may be able to manage supported squatting or kneeling.

There have been several cases of women who have decided to use epidural anaesthesia after a long or difficult labour and have then given birth squatting and enjoyed the second stage. However, you need to be helped into the squatting position by your attendants. In one recent case where the baby's heartbeat was dipping, it returned to normal as soon as she was upright and she gave birth completely naturally. In this case the midwife said that squatting saved the baby a forceps delivery.

Forceps or Ventouse

These are instruments used in the event of an emergency to help your baby out.

Forceps are like metal salad spoons with a hole in the middle that the obstetrician can insert on either side of the baby's head to help it out, and a ventouse or vacuum extractor attaches by suction to the baby's scalp to help extract the baby from your body.

Often the use of pain-relieving techniques such as epidurals weakens the power of the uterus so that forceps or ventouse are needed to extract the baby.

If you have an active birth you are less likely to need pain killers. By using standing, squatting or kneeling positions the need for forceps or ventouse is greatly reduced. Often after an active birth the midwife has commented that if the woman had been lying down she may well have needed the help of forceps. Occasionally an unusual presentation or a sudden rise in blood pressure or the baby being distressed would necessitate the use of forceps or ventouse. Although this has never been tried at the time of writing it seems that the 'all fours' position would be far better for these procedures than the usual reclining position, for the following reasons:

1. No compression on blood vessels so more oxygen to the baby.
2. Greater opening of the pelvic outlet.
3. Maximum relaxation of the perineum.
4. More efficient contractions.
5. Greater comfort to the mother.
6. Easier access.

Active Birth and Medication

Any drug you take in labour or pregnancy will filter through the placenta and enter your baby's bloodstream. None of them will do your baby any good. Opponents of natural childbirth say that they are not prepared to 'allow' nature to take its course unimpeded until it is proved to be safer than high technology. Despite this, almost all the drugs used in obstetrics have never been subjected to properly controlled, scientific evaluation and found to be safe regarding their effects on the development of the child (both at birth and in the long term). The research that has been done clearly indicates that when drugs are used routinely for normal childbirth, rather than as back-up treatment, they can often have damaging effects on the mother and child and on the bonding between them after birth.

When birth is active

- there is less need for drugs
- discomfort and pain are less
- the uterus functions better so artificial stimulants are not usually necessary
- labours are shorter
- the supply of oxygen to the baby is improved
- there is less need for forceps or ventouse
- the secretion of hormones which regulates the whole process is not disrupted.

Despite the readily available research on these findings the majority of women in this country are still confined to bed in labour, administered drugs and hooked up to a foetal monitor. Birth is still artificially induced and stimulated as soon as there is the slightest deviation from the average. This 'active management of labour' is usually done with the best of intentions to mother and child in the name of safety.

Undoubtedly there are always situations where medication helps to improve the experience and the safety factor, however, it is certainly debatable whether it does more harm than good when used routinely. Given that the majority of births are uncomplicated there is certainly not enough evidence in favour of the use of drugs to justify an overall policy.

Confining a women to bed in labour increases her need for pain-relieving drugs and artificial stimulants. Almost every woman given the freedom to move in labour has reported afterwards that when she lay down she was astonished how much more painful the contractions were.

'The only times the pain was extreme were those when I laid on my back for a pelvic examination by the midwife. I don't think I could have managed without any drugs if I had been lying down, as when I had to in the early stages it was unbearable.'

There are very few women who could go through labour on their backs without pain relief. Preventing a woman in labour from using her own instincts to find comfortable positions causes the need for pain killers and other drugs. The use of natural upright positions in childbirth throws a new light on the whole issue.

Some points for reflection

It is important to be able to make an informed choice when contemplating the use of drugs. The application of drugs is very well described in the literature on childbirth (see chapter 9, Recommended Reading) but often some of the well-known disadvantages are not mentioned.

Valium

● Causes amnesia (loss of memory) in 70 per cent of all women who use it and passes rapidly to the baby.

Pethidine

● Depresses the breathing response of the baby. A baby that has had a lot of pethidine may have difficulty establishing breathing and could suffer oxygen deficiency (particularly if the umbilical cord is cut immediately). An anti-depressant may be given to the baby to counteract the effects of the pethidine.

The baby may need to be resuscitated (given oxygen and helped to breathe). Pethidine also has the following reactions:

● It disturbs the baby's sucking reflex, often resulting in a sleepy baby and problems establishing breastfeeding which can last for several weeks, or result in failure.
● The pain relief is not very efficient unless given in large doses and then it often makes the mother drowsy, nauseous and less able to cope (particularly if it is mixed with a nausea suppressant).
● It works quite well as a muscle relaxant and can help dilation if given in small doses (25–50 mg).
● If given too late in labour (after 7 cm) the effect can be to ruin the second stage and will affect the baby more by remaining in its system for several days after the birth when it does not have the help of your body to clear away the waste products.
● If mother and baby are drowsy the bonding is disturbed.

Bupivacaine

- Used for epidurals and gives efficient pain relief from the waist down in most cases, without loss of consciousness. This is especially helpful for Caesareans where it would not need to be administered for a prolonged period and will have less effect on the baby. In this case it facilitates a good bonding as the mother is not unconscious.
- An epidural reduces the muscle tone of the uterus and bladder so that they function less efficiently. This increases the need for delivery by forceps by 20 per cent (using active upright postures for the second stage after tailing off the epidural at the end of the first stage would help to lower this percentage).
- The mother misses the pleasurable feelings as well as the pain, and may not be able to push her baby out spontaneously.
- Epidurals don't always work properly, sometimes they 'take' only down one side and are sometimes not easy to insert.
- There are after-effects such as headaches which can last for a week after the birth.
- Very occasionally a wrongly administered epidural can result in paralysis.
- Blood pressure is lowered which can result in less oxygen to the baby and long periods in the reclining position, necessary for an epidural, also diminish the oxygen supply.
- The lowering of blood pressure is useful in cases where it is dangerously high.
- Research shows that although the condition of the baby after an epidural is much better than with pethidine, epidural anaesthesia can cause either a nervous, jittery or a floppy, drowsy baby.
- The effects of this anaesthetic on the baby are still unknown, but it enters the baby's bloodstream and brain cells within minutes. Some recent research indicates that it could interfere with the development of the baby's brain and nervous system which is taking place during the period surrounding the labour and birth.

Gas and Oxygen (Entenox)

- Enters the baby's system and the effects are still under researched.
- Taken in large amounts it can make the mother feel nightmarish or detached 'out of her body'.
- A few whiffs in transition help some mothers to cope with the worst contractions.

Trilene

- Has a cumulative effect and can make mother and baby very drugged and sleepy.

Paracervical block

- Affects the baby immediately and makes its heartbeat slower which can result in death of the baby in extreme cases. For this reason it is not used very often in Britain.

Syntocin or Oxytocin drip

- Is used to stimulate uterine contractions and artificially induce or accelerate labour. The contractions are usually more powerful and closer together than in normal labour. If the contractions are very strong they can interrupt the normal blood flow to the placenta and this is more likely to result in foetal distress.
- There is a greater likelihood of the baby being born premature and needing special care, so that bonding will be disturbed. A premature baby is more at risk and is more likely to develop severe jaundice.
- The contractions are more violent, often have two peaks and are more difficult to cope with.
- A failed induction can result in a Caesarean section.

Post-natal depression rarely occurs when a woman has not taken any drugs and when the normal physiology of birth is not disturbed.

Conclusion

When there is a complication or life is at stake, obstetric intervention and medication provide a safety net. Often this can be combined with active birth and natural upright postures to the advantage of mother and baby. Used routinely for normal childbirth medication can cause problems and can have harmful effects both physically and psychologically.

Stillbirth

In the case of a stillbirth active labour has many advantages. It assists the mother to have a spontaneous birth without the use of drugs, which has proved to be very valuable as the mother feels she has gained something from the experience and may be able to use all her knowledge again in a future birth. She may not have a live baby, but she has had a labour. This can be a positive side of the experience. Also, if she delivers in the kneeling position, it gives her and her attendants time to prepare to see and hold the baby, which she will probably want to do. She will recover faster and feel physically well which will help her to cope with the emotional pain that is inevitable after such an experience.

Additionally, if the father of the baby is with her assisting her in the usual way, the experience will probably enhance their relationship and bring them closer together, which can only help.

'Looking back over my two pregnancies, my overwhelming impression is one of peaceful well-being. In both cases I started exercising regularly at about three months and experienced a growing satisfaction as I reached towards my body's potential. My first pregnancy sadly ended in a still-birth, but, on being encouraged to use all the positive elements gained from the classes, I tried for and achieved as good and natural a birth as possible. I feel sure that this helped enormously towards my ability to accept and live with the pain of the loss. How glad I was on giving birth to my second baby that I had had this first good experience.'

A Note to Birth Attendants

'My consultant's inate confidence in the normal workings of a healthy body was a real factor for calm and confidence both during my pregnancy and at the birth.'

If you are presented with this book by a woman who would like to put its teaching into practice we hope you will enjoy helping her to do so. It is hoped that the practice of active birth will help to make the atmosphere within the hospital more homely for those families who prefer, or for medical reasons choose, to have their babies in hospital. It is possible to combine some of the psychological advantages of home with the security of hospital by making a few basic changes. What is needed mainly is the right attitude towards the woman.

'There was a lovely Malaysian midwife and a girl student (whom I had already met). Both were very friendly and said 'do whatever you like'. Ditto the sister in charge of the labour ward, whom I knew from the time of Michael's birth since she had been on the postnatal ward –

she remembered and welcomed us, and offered to put a blanket on the floor if I wanted to carry on using my cushion.'

It is essential that the mother in labour should not be considered as a patient. The attendants should regard themselves as her guests, there to assist her in giving birth, which to her is a very special occasion in her sexual, social and emotional life. While carefully observing the progress of mother and baby the attendants should try not to disturb the natural process of the birth. Interference should be kept to an acceptable minimum to ensure safety. This means that both mother and midwife will rely more upon their instincts and intuition. Research has shown that whether at home or in hospital, when birth is regarded as natural and instinctive and interference is minimal, safety statistics are impressively better (i.e. in Holland and Pithiviers). With active birth the art of midwifery comes back into its own and midwives can become more spontaneous and flexible in their approach.

'I was taken straight into the labour ward and was given a big cushion so as to save my own from being soiled. Only one midwife was present and she let me do what I wanted, helping me squat, advising me on breathing and massaging me.'

The Birth Room

Here are some helpful ideas:

- Curtains which can be drawn to darken the room
- Dimmers on the lights
- A beanbag or pile of large cushions with attractive colourful covers
- A comfortable stool for squatting – perhaps a wooden birthstool.
- A comfortable armchair
- A casette tape recorder or record player (or suggestion to bring one's own)
- Sonicaid heart monitor
- A hot water bottle
- A kettle

Water is so helpful to mothers in labour that the birth room in hospital should include a bathroom and shower, or at least free access to those that already exist. Ideally a small pool, or double size bath, rather deeper than usual would be extremely helpful.

If a bed is used in a birth room it should not be too high or narrow. A low platform with a firm mattress is most comfortable. It should be remembered that furniture in a delivery room dictates how one should behave. If the first thing a women sees on entering the room is a delivery bed she immediately feels she ought to get into it, and is already a 'patient'.

It will help the mother greatly to feel at home if she is encouraged to use her body freely during labour and delivery and is free to give birth on the floor if she chooses to. A clean sheet with the usual sterile paper pad can be placed between her legs when the birth is imminent or, alternatively, a firm mattress could be placed on the floor.

Necessary checks on the dilation and foetal heart can be done with the minimum of discomfort and interruption to the mother in a position in which she is comfortable. It is important to bear in mind that a dilating cervix is also the most tender and vulnerable part of a woman's body and the seat of her deepest feelings. It would be of great comfort to some women and their husbands if they could bring a close woman friend or relative to the birth if they choose to do so. The emotional support would be doubled which would also help the staff. Some women would also very much like to have their other children present if circumstances allow. In some hospitals family birth rooms are being considered for this purpose.

Immediately after the birth it is helpful and encourages a good bonding situation if only the essential checking of the infant is done while in its mother's arms. Then the family should be left alone together for at least an hour and brought a cup of tea. The baby should be left naked but warmly wrapped up in a soft flannelette sheet so that the mother is free to explore her child. More detailed examination of the baby and stitching of tears can be done after this, if all is well.

Separation after a momentous occasion like a birth can be traumatic for a couple. If it were practical and possible for the father to stay for the first night this would help many families to enjoy their first hours together as a family and would have great psychological advantages.

'When everyone had gone and I lay bathed and clean between clean sheets with my man asleep on one side of me and litle babe in my arms I felt a supreme sense of peace and rightness with the world and the laws of nature.'

Working in a busy hospital where birth is a daily occurence it should be remembered that for the family concerned it is happening only once or a few times in a lifetime. The woman rightly needs to feel that she is the centre of what is happening, that this is her day. Her privacy and the profound and intimate nature of what she is experiencing should be respected at all times.

Midwifery is, to a large extent, a social profession – one is working with a family in childbirth or with a couple who are becoming a family. To the woman in labour the midwife is extremely important. If she feels her to be a friend, someone she can totally trust and relax with, the labour will progress better and will be a better experience for all concerned.

'Sue, our midwife, arrived very quickly, also a close friend. Their warmth and gentleness made us feel calm and very confident.'

Many of the factors to be considered are of a psychological and social nature. Naturally the primary concern to the midwife is the safe delivery of a healthy baby to a healthy mother. By encouraging mothers to give birth actively you will be helping them to achieve this in a way which is both safe and satisfying.

Should you wish to contact other professionals who have experience of attending women giving birth actively, see chapter 9 for some useful contacts and addresses.

The stretching exercises recommended in this book for mothers would also help attendants to be comfortable in kneeling and crouching positions in which they can assist a woman squatting (see Recommended Reading, chapter 9).

8
Stretching after the Birth

After giving birth to your child, your pelvic floor, uterus and vaginal area need to return to normal and your waist and belly need to regain their firmness and shape.

If you have stretched throughout your pregnancy your body's suppleness will have increased. While you were pregnant you had the benefit of hormones which your body produced to soften your joints. After the birth your hormone balance changes and if you continue to do the stretching exercises it will help you to maintain the flexibility and suppleness you have gained.

The after-birth stretches include exercises which tighten and firm your abdominal and pelvic floor muscles, others which strengthen your lower back and relax your neck and shoulders, and some for the muscles which support your breasts, helping to regulate the milk supply while you are breastfeeding. They will help you to recover your figure, and will help your uterus, vagina and pelvic floor to return to normal. They will give you plenty of vitality to enjoy your daily activities with your newborn child.

Motherhood makes considerable demands upon your body. You will need lots of energy and a sense of physical well-being for holding, carrying and lifting, for bending down, bathing and changing nappies, for breastfeeding and for playing with your baby.

In the first few months you need to adapt to a lot of changes, interrupted sleep and generally a whole new life-style with most of your activities centred around your child. Including some stretching in your day will help you to avoid fatigue and depression, will tune you in to your own body and will improve rest and sleep. You will learn to relax for yourself while enjoying your baby.

The stretching exercises that follow are intended for the first six months to a year after birth. The natural process of recovery after birth can take several months. Some women return to normal quicker than others, depending on the circumstances of the birth itself, weight gain during pregnancy and physical fitness.

The stretches are safe for everyone – start as soon after the birth as you feel ready and begin slowly with the first few movements, gradually adding the others one by one at your own pace. Your body will soon tell you if you are overdoing things. If your baby was born by Caesarean section then ask your doctor when you can begin exercising before you start. Take special care not to strain, particularly if you have backache, and follow the instructions carefully.

Useful tips

- Allow for the demands of motherhood on your time and energy. Do the stretching when you have time – when your baby is asleep or contented after a feed. Include your baby in the fun, and take things as they come. If your baby needs you, stop and carry on later.
- Be extra careful to avoid straining when bending or lifting as your lower back is very vulnerable after birth. When lifting something heavy bend your knees and keep your back straight, consciously keeping your shoulders and shoulder blades downwards and your buttocks firm. It is better to squat down with back straight to lift up your baby, your toddler, when cleaning, or gardening, than to stoop forward bending your back.

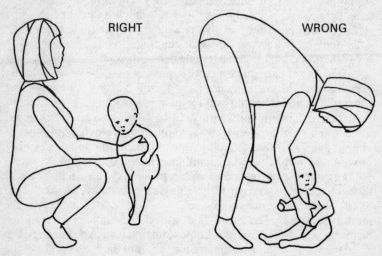

RIGHT   WRONG

● It is not a good idea to diet after you have had a baby, particularly if you are breastfeeding. You need rather more carbohydrates than normal to make milk. Eating a good balanced diet with three meals a day and plenty of fresh fruit and vegetables and whole grains and sufficient protein is very important.

● In the early days after birth it is a good idea to use a table for changing your baby to avoid bending your back.

● Sit on the floor a lot and attend to your baby with legs out-stretched and baby on your lap or between your legs. Sit up straight for breastfeeding or feed your baby lying down on your side with baby lying beside you.

● Wear flat-heeled shoes when carrying your baby and use a sling or baby-carrier when carrying for long periods of time.

1. Pelvic Floor Exercises

Note: Start with (a) the day after giving birth if you feel like it, after a few days add (b) but do not start (c) until three weeks after the birth.

a   Lie on your stomach on the floor, or in bed, face down with your arms straight and palms of your hands up by your sides. Tighten and relax your pelvic floor muscles. Repeat ten times (or more).

b   Now repeat, lifting up first one leg and tightening a few times, and then the other. You should feel this in the pelvic floor only. This has the same effect on your muscles as squeezing out a natural sponge in water. It brings in fresh blood, increases elasticity and improves muscle tone. This will promote healing if you have torn or have had an episiotomy.

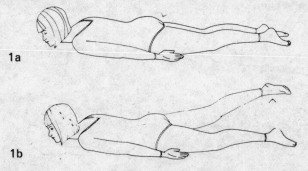

1a

1b

Pelvic floor exercises

c   Lie on your stomach on the floor. Tighten your buttocks and keep them tight. Lift up your head and lean lightly onto your elbows. Lift up your head and chest. Bring down your shoulders, don't hunch them. Keeping your buttocks tight, hold for a few seconds and then lie down and relax. Repeat several times. Take care to keep your shoulders down and don't remain in this position for a long period of time.

How you feel   You should feel the stretch in your abdomen and you will feel a pleasant sense of extension in your spine. If you keep your buttocks tight you shouldn't have any pain.

How you benefit   This exercise will stretch your abdominal muscles and gently extend your spine. It will help to tighten your pelvis and to develop strength in your lower back.

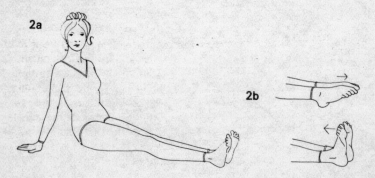

1c

2. Warm-up

This routine is a warm-up for the whole body – it will stimulate your circulation and loosen up your muscles and joints, ready for the stretching session.

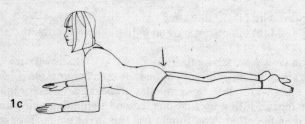

2a

2b

a   Sit up straight, legs together, stretched out in front of you. Place your hands just behind your buttocks, your weight resting on the palms. Keeping heels and feet in position, move toes only – backward, spreading them open and then forward. Repeat 8 times.

b   Bend your feet at the ankle joints. Point your toes, stretch them as far as possible from the body, then extend your heels and bring your toes up towards your body. Repeat 8 times.

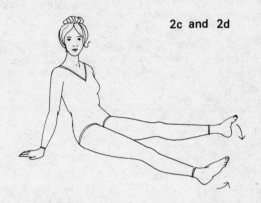

2c and 2d

c   Separate the legs slightly. Roll each leg loosely from the hips, first outwards and then inwards. Repeat several times.

d   Rotate your feet at the ankles, then move your feet in opposite circles, and reverse direction.

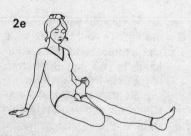

2e

e   Sit up straight with legs outstretched. Bend your left knee and lift the foot up onto your thigh, as close to your body as possible, and bounce the knee towards the ground. Hold for a minute or so then change to the other leg and repeat.

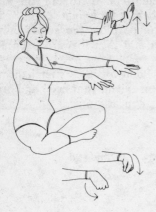

f Sit cross-legged, back straight and extend both arms at shoulder level.

● Bend wrists, move hands up and then down at wrists.

● Stretch fingers, hands wide, then clench fingers into a fist.

● Make fists of both hands and rotate at wrists in opposite circles. Reverse direction.

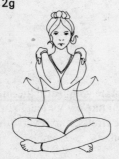

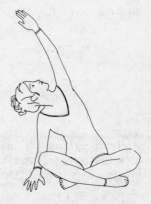

g Extend arms straight out at shoulder level, palms up. Drop your shoulders, keep your back straight. Bend your elbows and touch your shoulders with your finger tips. Rotate elbows in opposite circles. Make 8 circles and then reverse direction.

h Sit up straight with both legs drawn in to your body or with legs crossed and with your hands in your lap. Bend over to the left – left elbow towards the floor – right hand up. Come up and repeat to the right.

2i

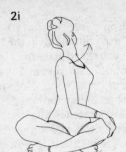

i   Sit up straight with your legs crossed. Stretch up, put your left hand on your right knee – your right hand palm down behind you and lift up – twist round to look over your right shoulder. Relax, face forward. Repeat to the left.

j   Head and Neck Exercises
●   Sit comfortably cross-legged, drop your shoulders and allow all tension to drop from your face.

Starting from the centre

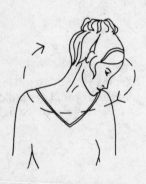

ii

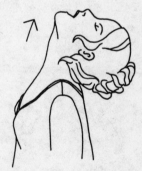

i   Let your head drop gently forward then slowly rotate your head, breathing slowly, allow the weight of your head to carry your head around in a full circle – to the side, front, side and back. Do three circles in each direction.

ii   Let your head hang back with mouth open wide. Hold for a few seconds, then bring your teeth together. Feel the stretch in your neck. Come up slowly.

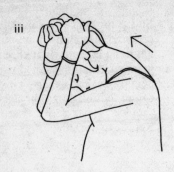

iii

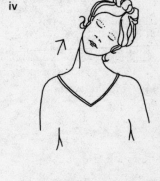

iv

iii Drop your head forward. Clasp your hands at the back of your head and gently bring your head down towards your breastbone. Hold for a few seconds breathing deeply. This stretches the back of your neck and upper back muscles. Come up slowly.

iv Lean your head over towards your left shoulder – feel the stretch down the side of your neck. Then reverse to the right.

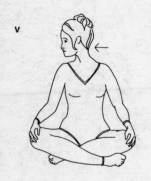

v

v Keeping your body still look round over your left shoulder and then reverse to the right.

3 On the wall

a Sit down sideways next to the wall so that your hip is touching the wall. Swing round so that your upper body is lying flat on the ground and your buttocks are close to or touching the wall. Bend your knees as if squatting and lift your arms up over your head. This is the resting position for this stretch.

b   Extend your arms over your head, palms up. When you do this
    make sure consciously that you do not raise your shoulders up.
    Keep your shoulder-blades down as you raise your arms
    overhead. You should feel the stretch in your shoulders and chest.
c   Now, slowly, keeping shoulders down and arms straight, lift up
    your arms to 90 degrees and then slowly lower them to your sides,
    palms down. Relax, then lift your arms up again and place them on
    the ground above your head, palms up.
    Breathe in as you lift your arms up, breathe out when you lower
    them. Repeat 6 times, end with arms up. Breathe naturally and
    relax.
d   Now, stay in this position, bring your hands together above your
    head and with arms straight and keeping them on the ground,
    bring them round to your sides to describe a full circle. Relax and
    then bring your arms back up to behind your head. Breathe out
    when you lower your arms, breathe in when you bring them up.
    End on an out-breath with hands by your sides.

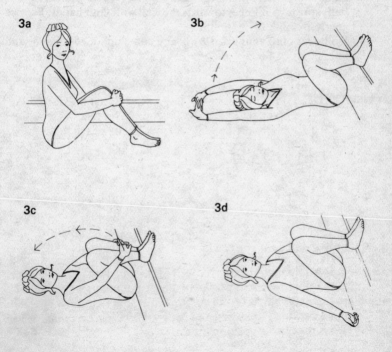

How you benefit   This stretch relaxes the shoulders and the muscles which support your breasts and opens the chest, while gently strengthening your lower back. It helps you to breathe well. This exercise will help to regulate the milk supply if you are breastfeeding.

Legs Apart on the Wall

e   Straighten your legs, keeping your knees tight and hold for a few seconds until you are used to this position.

f   Allow your legs to drop open as far as they can keeping your knees tight and extending your heels. Put your arms back over your head.

Now, bend your knees and straighten, bend and straighten several times. Then keep your knees straight, point your toes and then the opposite, bring them in towards your body, extending your heels. Do this several times and then hold the position for five minutes or more breathing deeply and relaxing into it. Now repeat the arm exercises 3a–3d.

g   Bend your knees, bring the soles of your feet together, close to your body, press your knees towards the wall with your hands. Bounce gently.

Roll over onto your side slowly and come up on your hands and knees.

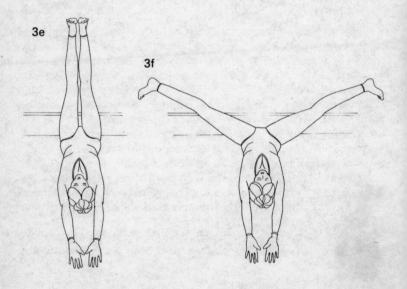

3e

3f

3g

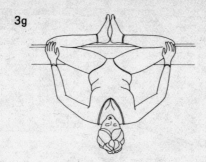

How you benefit   These stretches lengthen and relax the inner thigh muscles, strengthen the back and relax the upper chest and shoulders. They will help you to maintain the flexibility you gained during pregnancy and improve your circulation, making you feel more energetic. This routine is beneficial for varicose veins and haemorrhoids and will promote healing of the pelvic floor after birth. Your baby will enjoy being held up in the air or bouncing on your knees in this position.

4   Butterfly

a   Sit with your back straight. Bring the soles of your feet together as close to your body as possible. Put your hands behind you, palms down, close to your buttocks to help keep your back straight – or else clasp your feet with your hands. Make small 'butterfly' movements with your legs to loosen your hip joints. Keep your back straight. Lift up from your tailbone – don't allow your pelvis to slump back. You can use this as a sitting position.

b   Bring your feet forward – a little further from your body – bounce your knees. Then bring them in close to your body and bounce.

c   Now spread your legs wide apart as possible. Keep your back straight. Point your toes and then hook them back – extending your heels and bringing toes towards your body – repeat several times. This can be used as a sitting position when playing with your baby.

d   End up by bending your knees bringing the soles of your feet together – drawing them close to your body again. Bounce and relax.

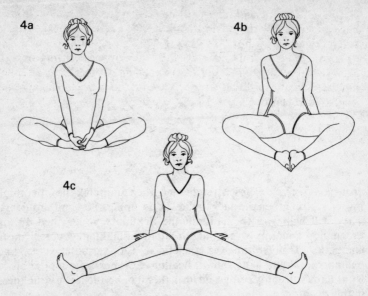

How you feel In this position you should feel the stretch mainly in the groin and hip joints and you may also feel it in your knees and ankles.

How you benefit This stretch maintains good suppleness in the hip joints. It tones up the pelvic muscles, helping the uterus to return to shape and enables a good circulation of blood to this area. This exercise will help to promote healing after the birth in the case of a tear or episiotomy.

5 Pelvic Tuck-ins

a Sit between your feet, ankles turned out and toes pointing towards each other, or else sit on your heels. With knees apart and moving from the hips, come forward onto your hands, keeping spine and arms straight.

b Now breathe in as you come forward, bringing your weight onto your hands and tightening your buttock muscles as you tuck in your pelvis.

Hold for a few seconds then let go on an outbreath and relax bringing your weight back onto your knees. Repeat several times building up a rhythm.

This movement will help to strengthen your buttocks and lower back and to firm up the pelvic organs. If you have backache then do this several times throughout the day.

You can follow this exercise with the Japanese sitting or Frog exercises from 'Stretching for Pregnancy' (see chapter 2, no. 3), to help maintain the flexibility of your pelvic joints, to prevent backache and improve circulation.

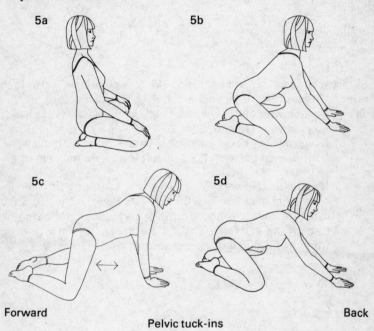

5a

5b

5c

5d

Forward

Back

Pelvic tuck-ins

6   Shoulder Stretch

Sit between your feet, or on your heels, knees together and back straight. Drop your shoulders and clasp your hands in your lap in front of you. If you can, reverse them turning your palms out. Breathe in and keeping your elbows straight, stretch up and lift your arms above your head, hold for a second and keep breathing then come down on an outbreath. Repeat several times.

This exercise helps to tone up your breasts, opens and relaxes your chest and promotes good breathing.

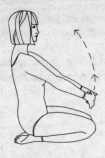

Shoulder stretch

7   Pelvic Lift

Sit between your feet, ankles turned out, toes pointing towards each other. Alternatively, sit on your heels. Keep your knees together.

7a   Tighten your buttock muscles and lean back onto your hands keeping your arms straight.

Keep your buttocks tight, tuck in your pelvis so that your pubic bone lifts up in front. Hold for a few seconds and then let go. Repeat several times.

7b   If you can sit between your feet then you can follow this exercise with 'lying back between the feet' (see chapter 2, no. 6). Take care to introduce your body to this very gradually following the instructions carefully. The full posture should only be done from the third month after the birth.

7a   7b

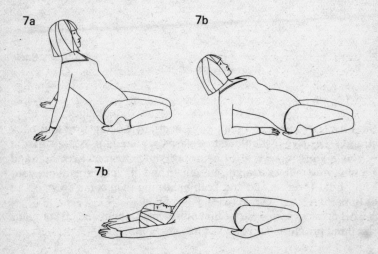

7b

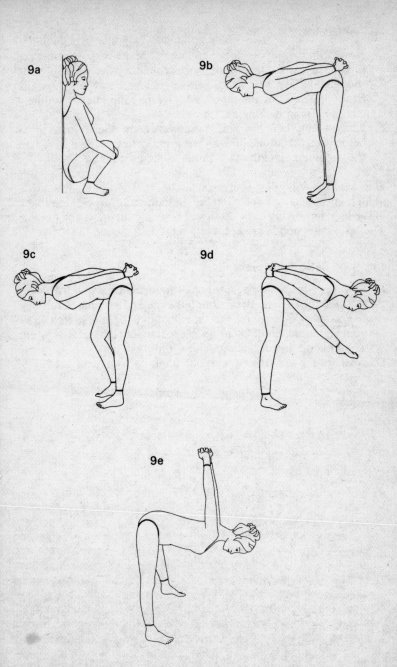

9a

9b

9c

9d

9e

d   Now, stand with your feet 3 feet apart. Make sure your feet are turned in rather than out, open your chest and drop your shoulders. Clasp your hands behind your back and bend forward from the hips on an outbreath. Keep your back absolutely straight. Hang or bounce. Come up.

e   Clasp hands behind back. Elbows straight. Bend forward as before, only this time lift up your arms until you feel a stretch in the shoulders. Hold for a second, come down.

How you benefit   This routine helps to maintain flexibility of the ankles, knees and hips and stretches the hamstring muscle at the back of the legs, improving circulation and relieving tiredness and fatigue. The last one is good for shoulders, chest and breasts too.

10   Side Bend and Twist

a   Stand up straight with your back supported by a wall with your feet one foot apart. Bend your left knee and keeping your body flat on the wall, bend over to the left until you feel a stretch down your right side, hold. Come up. Repeat to the right, breathing out as you bend down. Repeat several times.

b   Now try the same thing with one hand up over your head.

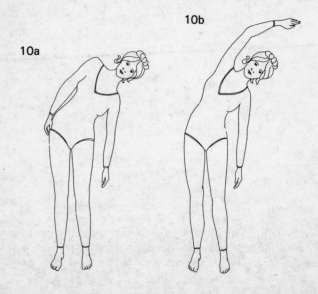

10b

10a

c Now try the same thing clasping your hands together over your head, with elbows straight.

d **Spiral Twist** Stand up straight with feet one foot apart. Bend your knees a little, tighten your buttocks and turn around so that your spine turns and your chest faces the wall while your hips face frontwards. Keep your shoulders down and place your hands on the wall with elbows bent, hold for a second. Then relax and repeat on the other side. Repeat several times.

e Stand with feet 3 feet apart with your back supported by a wall. Turn your left foot out parallel to the wall. Turn your right foot in, in the same direction. Place your hands on your hips and keep your spine against the wall. Be aware of your head as a continuation of one straight line from your tailbone. Keeping your hips flat against the wall, bend over from the hips towards your left foot. Hold and slowly come up. Repeat to the other side.

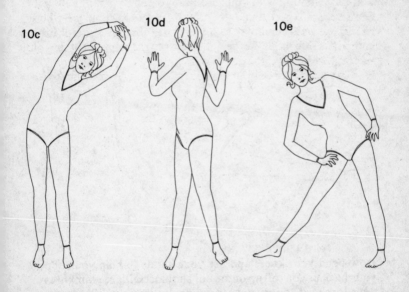

10c   10d   10e

How you benefit This routine helps you to regain your waistline and stretches the side muscles. The twisting exercise also helps to lubricate the spine and strengthen your back.

You can also benefit from the reclining twist (see chapter 2, no.15). It will strengthen your back and help restore your waistline. The shoulder stretch (chapter 2, no.7) is also very beneficial and will relax your shoulders and open your chest.

11   Shoulder Stand

a   Lie down on the floor on your back with your legs stretched out in front of you and a chair behind your head. Place your arms at your sides, hands palms down.

11a

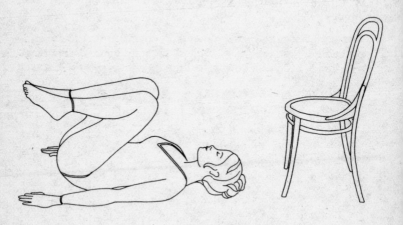

b   Now bend your knees and use your hands to help you support your back as you roll up onto your shoulders. Place your knees on your forehead and try to keep your spine straight, lifting up your hips. Your weight is carried by your neck and shoulders. Support your back with your hands. Hold for a second and then roll back down slowly, vertebrae by vertebrae, keeping your knees bent and your arms, hands palms down, by your side.

11b

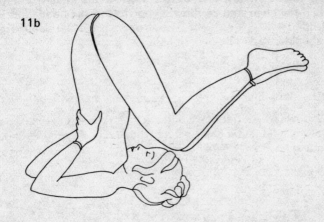

c   Repeat, only this time after bending your knees and rolling up, straighten your legs to 90 degrees, keeping your buttocks tight and lifting up. Bend your knees and roll down in the same way.

11c

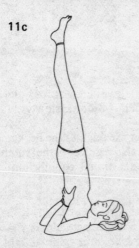

d   Repeat, only this time, lower your legs over your head one at a time, keeping your knees straight until your feet rest on the chair behind your head. Hold for a few seconds, then bend your knees and roll down slowly in the same way. After a while you may not need the chair and can lower your feet to the floor, over your head.

11d

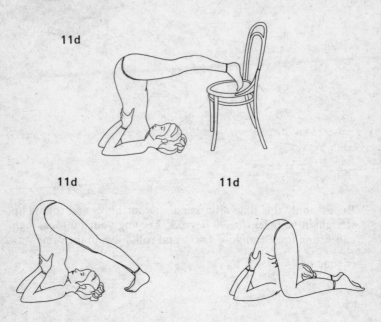

11d

11d

After (d) try also bending your knees and placing them beside your ears. Hold and then roll down slowly.

How you benefit   This exercise releases the neck and shoulders and has a very calming effect. It also regularises the secretion of hormones, which helps to maintain emotional equilibrium and to promote breastfeeding.

12   Relaxation

● Lie down flat on the floor with legs apart and arms spread out. Hands, palms up. Relax deeply letting go each part of your body in turn.

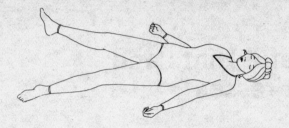

- Breathe deeply, concentrating on the outbreath and pause between each breath so that you are aware of a still space between each breath.
- Feel your belly rise when you breathe in and fall when you breathe out.
- Relax completely – your whole body should be limp and heavy. Allow your thoughts to pass by – try to keep your attention focused on the outbreath.

Spend five or ten minutes in total relaxation after stretching or at any other time of day.

9
Useful Hints and Addresses

Alcohol

Taken in excess alcohol can harm your baby. The occasional glass of wine is all right. In labour alcohol will stop contractions – it is used to prevent threatened miscarriage.

Anaemia

If you are anaemic your baby may suffer because less oxygen is carried to the placenta. You are also more likely to bleed heavily after birth and are more prone to infection.

Eat plenty of protein foods, leafy green vegetables, dried apricots and take vitamins B, B12 and C. A tonic such as Floradix which contains absorbable iron (or else iron tablets prescribed by your doctor) would help. Floradix is available from health food stores. It can also be helpful to consult a herbalist and/or homoeopath, as there are remedies which can help anaemia.

Artificial rupture of membranes (ARM/Amniotomy)

This is done by inserting an instrument like a crochet hook through the cervix and breaking the membranes which surround the baby. The result will be that the amniotic fluids drain away and the contractions usually intensify. This is sometimes done to induce or accelerate labour and in some hospitals is a routine procedure on admission.

Normally the membranes break spontaneously before, during or at the moment of birth. Most commonly they break towards the end of the first stage. There is usually no need to rupture artificially – in fact there are some disadvantages to doing so:

- The wedge of fluid between the baby's head and the contracting uterus is lost so there is more pressure on the head and on the cord from the powerful contractions of the uterus. This can cause a decrease in the flow of blood to and from the baby and there is some evidence which indicates that the baby's heart-rate slows down slightly.
- There is also increased risk of infection as the intact membranes and the amniotic fluid provide protection.
- The contractions can suddenly be much stronger and more painful after an ARM, and it can be very difficult to cope with this rapid increase in intensity.
- The baby is probably more comfortable with water between its body and the powerful contractions of the uterus.

However, sometimes amniotomy is carried out because there are signs of foetal distress (such as irregularity of the heart-beat), and it will help to assess the condition of the baby by checking the colour of the water. If the water contains meconium (the first bowel movement of the baby) it is stained green or brown. This can be an indication that the baby is distressed. In order to attach a scalp electrode heart monitor it is necessary to rupture the membranes first.

Early Rupture of the Membranes

If your membranes break before labour starts there is increased risk of infection as you do not have the protective barrier of the sealed water bag around the baby. Usually infection does not occur and contractions will start up after a few hours, but sometimes it can take longer. If contractions have not started after 12 hours the risk of infection is greater.

To prevent infection you must keep very clean, washing down after each visit to the toilet. Don't lie down in the bath – rather take a shower or kneel upright in the bath to wash down. (It's all right to lie in the water if you do have contractions.)

Garlic tablets and vitamin C will have a naturally antibiotic effect and prevent infection without harming you or the baby. Take 7–8 garlic capsules and 1 gm vitamin C every 2–3 hours till you go into labour. The garlic does tend to 'repeat' on one so perhaps your partner should take a few too!

Homoeopathic caulophyllum may help to start the contractions.

Bleeding

Sometimes in the first three months slight bleeding or spotting can occur at the time you would normally have had your period. This is usually no problem. However, as bleeding of any sort in pregnancy could indicate a possible problem you should rest in bed, stop exercising and inform your doctor immediately. A small amount of spotting or bleeding is usually no cause for concern. If you have a serious problem with bleeding it is probably better not to do any stretching at all, to be on the safe side. There are homoeopathic and herbal remedies which may be helpful.

Blood Pressure

Blood pressure is the term which refers to the pressure exerted by the blood on the walls of the blood vessels. The systolic pressure is measured when the heart is contracted and is pushing the blood out and the diastolic pressure is the pressure in the arteries when the heart is relaxed between beats. It is written systolic/diastolic, like this for instance: 115/70. Normal systolic pressure ranges from 100–125 with some variation and the diastolic is usually between 60 and 80.

Eating a good diet, with enough protein and stretching during pregnancy will help to maintain normal blood pressure. Your blood pressure will be checked throughout pregnancy and labour. A slight rise in b/p is fairly common at the end of pregnancy but if the diastolic figure in the reading rises by as much as 15 you are considered to have hypertension. This need not necessarily, but can be, a symptom of pre-eclampsia or toxaemia which is a possible complication of pregnancy.

The symptoms of pre-eclampsia in its mild form are high blood pressure with oedema (swelling) and protein in the urine. If you have toxaemia then it is safest to have your baby in hospital. Sometimes, with bed-rest and good diet, mild pre-eclampsia will improve. The latest research reveals that it is not wise to cut out salt but more helpful to eat extra protein. The problem here is that you feel perfectly well but all the same the condition does need attention.

Very rarely these days does pre-eclampsia lead to eclampsia. The symptoms are headaches, dizziness, irritability, nausea, visual disturbances and pain in the upper abdomen.

If there is protein in the urine it can be a sign of failure of the placenta and may result in premature labour or deprivation to the baby, which is why medical experts prefer to induce labour when there is persistent pre-eclampsia.

Sometimes hypertension is related to emotional stress but not necessarily. There are homoeopathic and herbal remedies which help high blood pressure.

If you are confined to bed it will help to get up every few hours and do a little very relaxed stretching for half an hour and then return to bed. This will help you to exercise your body, keep up your morale, while possibly lowering your blood pressure.

Breasts

To prepare your breasts during pregnancy simply massage them with a little almond oil (or any other vegetable oil) after your bath. Don't use soap on your nipples as this tends to dry up all the natural oils. Do not wear a bra – or only a cotton one. The National Childbirth Trust (see addresses) stock 'mava' bras which are ideal for maternity wear. In the days after the birth when your breasts fill up with milk you will find one of these very helpful.

Breastfeeding

It is important to learn about breastfeeding and babycare before you actually go into labour. An active birth, followed by a good bonding in the first hour after birth is the foundation of a good breastfeeding relationship. When the natural physiology is undisturbed then one event will flow into another quite naturally. However, there can be problems with establishing breastfeeding in the early days and sometimes one needs good advice quickly. Contact the La Leche League or your local NCT breastfeeding counsellor while you are still pregnant.

Recommended reading:
The experience of breastfeeding by Sheila Kitzinger, and *Touching* by Ashley Montague.

Breech position

See chapter 7, Unusual Presentations.

Constipation

The best remedy is squatting, lots of it. Also eat bran and dried fruit such as prunes. There are herbal and homoeopathic remedies too.

Cramp

This occurs in the legs and no one knows for sure what causes it, but lots of stretch no. 10 (chapter 2) usually helps to eradicate it. When seized by a cramp, extend your heel, bringing your toes up towards your body and rub the muscles vigorously. Sometimes when you begin stretching, cramps in the foot are common in the kneeling positions. Eventually, with practice this will pass.

Drugs

See chapter 7, Active Birth and Medication.

Due date

As some women have longer or shorter menstrual cycles, some have longer or shorter pregnancies. Your due date is only the estimated average – two or even three weeks either way is not uncommon. Late for dates alone (without any other sign of complications) is not a good reason for inducing labour. It is a good reason for careful observation and for testing the placental function (see Placental Insufficiency). Similarly, if you go into labour two or three weeks before your date your baby will not necessarily be premature.

Eating in labour

When you are in labour your body tends to want to empty itself of its contents. It is not a good idea to eat large meals or indigestible foods. On the other hand if you have a long labour you are going to need some food to sustain you or you may become exhausted. When this happens you feel very low and wasted and labour can cease to progress well. Medically it is known as being 'ketotic'. If your urine is tested and contains acetone then this is a sign of ketosis.

Most hospitals do not allow a woman in labour to eat anything at all (in case you need a Caesarian), but prefer to attach you to a glucose drip to avoid ketosis. The disadvantage is that this usually means that you are immobile and restricted to the reclining position, and also you may be hungry! Ketosis can be avoided by the following:

- In early labour eat a light meal, such as a slice of toast, an egg, some yoghurt with wheatgerm and honey, or some soup.
- Have some nourishing, but very liquid soup around and take a few spoonfuls every now and then. Miso soup, or chicken soup are ideal. Take some to hospital in a thermos flask.
- Have some form of sugar every now and then, such as a spoonful of honey in boiling water, or herb tea, or some red grape or apple juice. If you do become slightly ketotic take some glucose tablets and drink sips of fruit juice (not citrus fruits) between every contraction.
- Make sure your husband or partner has some food to take into hospital as he is unlikely to be offered any in a busy labour ward.

Emergency birth

If you are alone with a woman who is about to give birth and are unable to reach midwife or doctor then:

- Try to relax and stay calm. Take a few deep breaths with good long outbreaths. Surprise births are usually completely straightforward.
- Comfort the mother and if there is time reassure her by holding her for a minute or two. Suggest that she go on all fours on her hands and knees or into the knee-chest position, while you get everything ready. Give her a large cushion if there is one.

This will help to slow down the contractions a little and will help her to feel more in control and will calm her.

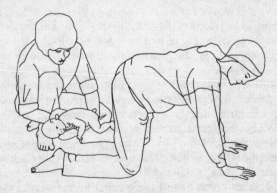

All fours position

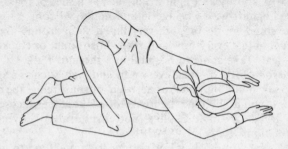

Knee-chest position

- Get some clean towels, sheets, newspapers, or coats and a duvet if possible to cover the mother and baby, also a towel or soft jumper to wrap the baby in.
- Close all windows and try to warm the room as mother and baby need to be kept very warm.
- Boil a kettle and switch it off while you wash your hands really well. Get a glass of water, a bowl and a toilet roll or cotton wool.
- Go back to the mother, massage her lower back gently and calmly. Give her sips of water and plenty of reassurance. Place a clean sheet, or towel or newspaper underneath her and have some more handy. Have something nearby to wrap the baby in. Place it near a heater to warm up.
- Once you can give her your undivided attention she can stay in that position or else squat against a cushion or beanbag (she could use a low stool), or one or two large books covered over with plastic bag and towel if there is time. Any position she chooses will be all right.
- Allow nature to take its course. Encourage her to take her time and open up, and give way to what is happening inside her. If she panics, breathe deeply with her concentrating on the OUT-BREATH. Suggest that she breathe the baby out rather than push forcefully.
- If she is nauseous or sick don't worry. This is quite normal and is just part of the expulsive reflex.
- If any faeces come out of the mother's anus wipe it clean with toilet paper – away from the vagina.

- The baby may come out in one contraction or else over several. Receive the baby without pulling. Allow her uterus to do all the work, just 'catch' the baby. Allow the head to hang down a little as this will help the shoulders to come out.
- If the cord is around the baby's neck this is quite common and perfectly normal, simply try to loosen it a little with your finger. Don't pull on it as this could dislodge the placenta. Once the baby is born simply free the cord from the baby's neck.
- If the mother is squatting, hold the baby face down between her feet for a half a minute or so to drain the fluids and then let the mother pick him up in her arms.
- If she is on all fours then receive the baby. Hold it face down for a moment and then pass through her legs to the mother.

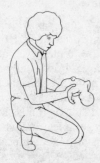

- The mother should sit upright with her baby. If a lot of fluid has come out of her then she could possibly move over to a clean sheet or towel.
- Keep them both warm with duvet, towel, coats, whatever you have handy. The baby's head should be covered too.
- Sit down and enjoy a few peaceful moments with mother and baby. Encourage the mother to place her baby to the breast as this will stimulate the uterus to contract. Don't leave the mother alone in the house.
- Telephone for a midwife or doctor to come round.
- If the placenta comes out between the mother's legs place it in a bowl. Don't cut the cord as it will stop pulsating and clamp itself spontaneously.
- After the placenta is out the uterus should contract down and feel like a grapefruit. If it doesn't then you or the mother should massage her belly firmly to stimulate the uterus to contract.

- If you have some, give the mother some arnica or rescue remedy and perhaps a cup of tea with sugar or honey.
- Use the previously boiled and cooled water from the kettle to wash the mother's genital area, although it is best if she can squat over a bowl of warm water and do it herself. Then give her a sanitary towel or clean towel to place between her legs and a pair of clean knickers.

If the birth takes place in a taxi or some unusual place, then your priorities are to stay relaxed, reassure the mother, catch the baby and keep them both warm.

Fluid retention (oedema)

This is seen as a slight swelling or puffiness in the ankles and fingers and is fairly common in late pregnancy. Homoeopathy is very helpful in reducing oedema (the remedy is nat. mur. but consult a homoeopath for the dosage). It is usually nothing to worry about if your blood pressure and urine are all right, but you should report the matter to your doctor. As soon as the birth is over the oedema disappears. Don't cut out salt or fluids, but do eat well – plenty of protein, fresh fruit and vegetables, and whole grains. If the puffiness is severe it may be a sign of pre-eclampsia (see blood pressure).

Exercise no. 4 (see chapter 2), *Legs apart on the wall*, will help to reduce the swelling. You could do it several times a day and keep your feet up when relaxing.

Foetal distress

This happens when a baby is not getting enough oxygen and is usually indicated by the following two symptoms:

1. A baby is distressed when its heart rate falls or rises and is consistently lower or faster than the normal limits of 120–160 beats per minute.
2. When a baby lacks oxygen in labour its anal sphincter tends to relax and some of the first bowel movement (meconium) passes into the amniotic fluid, turning it brown or green. Meconium staining is not always a sign of distress but coupled with irregularity of the heartbeat it is very likely that the baby is in

trouble. If the baby inhales meconium into its lungs it can congest the lungs and cause respiratory problems.

It is not necessary to rupture the membranes to check if the amniotic fluid is meconium-stained unless there is a consistent irregularity of heartbeat.

Some causes of foetal distress
- Compression of the major internal blood vessels (as in the reclining position).
- Prolonged labour.
- Premature induction.
- Large doses of analgesic such as pethidine which depress the mother's nervous system, diminishing the flow of blood to and from the baby.
- Placental misfunction.
- Prolapse, entanglement or compression of the cord.
- Diabetes or toxaemia of the mother.

Ways to avoid or alleviate foetal distress
a Keep active and upright during labour.
b If the heartbeat of the baby is irregular try changing positions to vertical or kneeling.
c If foetal distress occurs in the second stage then the upright standing squat is the best way to get the baby born quickly.
d It may be necessary to use forceps, ventouse, episiotomy or Caesarean section to help a distressed baby.

Haemorrhoids (piles)

These are like varicose veins which occur in the anus. Do 50 anal tightening exercises (like pelvic floor exercises only concentrate on the anal muscles) in the morning before you get out of bed, and 50 at night before you go to sleep. Consult a homoeopath and make sure you aren't constipated. For extreme or protruding haemorrhoids don't do full squatting – do the dictionary squat instead. Try homoeopathic ointments or compresses of calendula or witch hazel. Ask your doctor's advice too.

Headaches

These can occur more frequently in pregnancy. Eat well, get plenty of sleep and don't overdo things. If you feel a headache coming on do the head and neck exercises (chapter 2, stretch no. 1) concentrating on the forward part. Do some stretches to loosen your shoulders (chapter 2, no. 7). Breathe deeply and relax in a darkened room for a while. You should inform your doctor if you have severe or frequent headaches.

Heartburn

This is very common in pregnancy and is usually caused by a softening of the valve between your oesophagus and your stomach by hormones (the same hormones that soften your joints), so that your food tends to rise up. Eat several small meals rather than one large one and avoid acidic foods. Try stretches no. 4 and no. 7. Make some umeboshi juice: Take 3 umeboshi plums (from a health food store) boil in a pint of water and keep the juice in the fridge. Drink a little when you have heartburn.

Herbs

Herbal teas
Especially good for pregnancy. You can mix them together to make a taste you enjoy or have them separately.

   Raspberry leaf (good for uterus)
   Camomile (soothing)
   Peppermint (stimulating)
   Rosehip (vitamin c)

Herbal bath for after birth
A soothing healing antiseptic miracle for perineal tears, grazes or episiotomies.

   Ingredients   Shepherds Purse
               Uva Ursi
               Comfrey
               6 whole heads garlic (Enough for 2 lots)

Method Take three heads of garlic. Do not peel but prick all over with a fork. Put in a large saucepan with a generous handful of each of the herbs. Fill up with water and bring to the boil. Simmer gently for ½–¾ hour. Squeeze the juice out of the garlic with a fork or masher and then cool it. Strain the liquid into a large jar. Put the whole lot into a warm bath and sit in it for a while. Use once or twice daily at least. (Use Calendula tincture as well and put some in water to wash yourself after you urinate.)

Herbs available from: Culpeppers (Flask Walk, Hampstead)
Haelen Centre (Park Road, Crouch End)

and many other good herb and health food stores.

Home birth

Finding out about home birth

First ask your GP if he/she does home births. If not then ask for referral to a GP who will. If there isn't one contact the Area Nursing Officer (at the city or county health department) to get a list of GPs who do home confinements. Also tell the Community Nursing Officer that you want a home birth and ask her advice.

If that fails write to your Community Health Council Area Nursing Officer and Family Practitioner Committee (addresses from the health department). By law a midwife, called when you are in labour at home, must attend. Also try the Birth Centre, ARMS, AIMS and SSHC (see Useful Addresses).

Homoeopathy

Homoeopaths recommend certain remedies for pregnancy and labour. The following are generally recommended but consult a homoeopath for any special problems.

The Pregnancy Programme devised by John Damonte, a famous homoeopath, is suitable for general use by any woman who is pregnant and wishes to ensure that she and her baby will be fit and strong throughout pregnancy, delivery and breastfeeding.

It is not necessary to take iron tablets if you take this programme.

2nd and 6th month: CALC FLUOR 6x + MAG PHOS 6x + FERR PHOS 6x
3rd and 7th month: CALC FLUOR 6x + MAG PHOS 6x + NAT MUR 6x
4th and 8th month: CALC FLUOR 6x + NAT MUR 6x + SILICA 6x
5th and 9th month: CALC FLUOR 6x + FERR PHOS 6x + SILICA 6x.

Amongst other things, CALC FLUOR promotes elasticity of vessels and tissues, diminishing the risk of ruptures and lessening the chances for episiotomy; MAG PHOS helps to deal with heartburn and digestive problems; FERR PHOS stimulates the process of absorption of iron preventing anaemia; NAT MUR helps to keep a proper balance in the fluid distribution, while SILICA strengthens both the mother's and the baby's bones and sinews.

Homoeopathy can help with many of the minor complaints and discomforts of pregnancy such as nausea, water retention, heartburn, high blood pressure etc., as well as existing chronic conditions, but it is necessary to consult a practitioner before taking remedies (see Useful Addresses).

There are a few remedies which are helpful to all women in labour which anyone can safely take without consulting a homoeopath. They do not clash with other medication or drugs, and are of benefit to the baby as well.

Arnica
Reduces bruising, shock, fear and bleeding. It will also help to soften internal tissues, and prevent swelling: Take one dose of Arnica 200 at the onset of labour. During the birth take another dose whenever necessary (if necessary at all) and after the birth one dose per day until all discomfort is gone.

Bach Rescue Remedy
A composition of five flower essences, and is very effective when pain or panic becomes overwhelming during labour, without dulling the vivid and intense experience of delivery. Take 10 drops in a little water. This remedy is particularly helpful in transition.

Caulophyllum
This is a remedy which tones and relaxes the uterus. Take one once a week (30x strength) for 2–3 weeks before your expected date. It will prepare the uterus for labour. Caulophyllum or Cimifuga can help during labour if contractions stop or are irregular. Consult a homoeopath about the dosage.

Calendula Mother Tincture
This remedy is a healing antiseptic – use instead of synthetic antiseptics. Put 10 drops in an egg cup of warm water that has been boiled, to clean baby's cord. Put 10 drops in a bowl of warm

previously boiled water to bathe stitches (do this after you urinate in the days after the birth). Use Calendula diluted or neat for sore nipples. Apply neat, using a warm sterilised natural sponge, to stitches in the days after birth.

Use throughout childhood to treat infection, cuts, grazes and wounds. There is also Calendula talcum powder – useful for the cord and for drying baby's creases.

Common teething problems may be relieved by chamomilla (in the potency prescribed by your Homoeopath). Other common problems such as cholic and rashes may be helped homoeopathically. There are soothing and healing homoeopathic ointments such as Hypercal or Calendula and a wonderful ointment for burns which should be in every medicine chest.

Homoeopathic remedies can be obtained from some chemists and health food stores or a homoeopathic pharmacy such as A. Nelson & Co., 215–233 Coldharbour Lane, London SW9 BRU (by post), or their main branch in Duke Street, London.

There is a booklet on Homoeopathy in Pregnancy and Childhood with notes on diet, published by the Society of Homoeopaths, 101 Sebastian Avenue, Shenfield, Brentwood, Essex, CM15 8PP.

Inducing labour

See chapter 7. Labour usually happens when the time is right. More natural ways of inducing labour are: (a) Love-making, there is natural prostoglandin in semen which softens the cervix, and the relaxation and orgasm may help to start you off. (b) Exercise. (c) An enema. (d) Castor oil (must be prescribed by your doctor). This will cause diarrhoea which may stimulate the labour. (e) Go out and enjoy yourself – have a glass or two (not more) of wine.

Insomnia

Is there anything worrying you which is keeping you awake? Have a hot bath and do your stretching before going to bed. Drink camomile tea in the evenings. Consult a homoeopath.

Internal Examinations

See chapter 7.

Iron

See anaemia.

Jaundice

About half of all babies get mild jaundice in the first week of life. They look a little suntanned. It is caused by the baby's liver still being a little immature and unable to cope completely with the breakdown of bilirubin. Premature babies are more prone to jaundice. The baby should be put to the breast a lot as it needs the fluid. Sunlight will be helpful and maybe a sip of previously boiled water on a teaspoon periodically.

Ketosis

See Eating in labour.

Miscarriage

If you have sudden bleeding, pain in the abdomen or contractions go to bed, phone your doctor immediately and have a drink of brandy or whisky.

Monitoring

See chapter 7.

Morning Sickness (nausea)

Starting stretching every day and consult a homoeopath. Homoeopathic remedies such as petrol or sepia can be very helpful but you need the right one for your constitution. Eat small meals frequently and have some milk and a cracker as soon as you wake up in the morning. Morning sickness usually passes by the end of the first three months.

Oedema

See Fluid retention.

Orgasm

In pregnancy love-making and orgasm are as beneficial to you as ever. Some women do not want to make love when they are pregnant and some do more than ever. Gentle love-making can't harm your baby. Try different positions, i.e. kneeling on all fours, lying side by side, penetration from behind etc., to avoid any weight on your belly. Towards the end of pregnancy you may find more shallow penetration or masturbation more comfortable.

This is a great time to experiment and try some new ideas!

Piles

See Haemorrhoids.

Placental Insufficiency

To avoid this eat well during your pregnancy. If this is suspected then ask for tests to be done.

The oestriol test examines the amount of oestrogen in your blood and urine. If the oestrogen is high then it's possible that your placenta isn't functioning well. If you have no other symptoms other than being past your due date placental insufficiency is unlikely.

Posterior Presentation

See chapter 7, Unusual presentations.

Rhesus Factor

The Rh factor is found in the red blood cells.

Most people are Rh positive (Rh+), 15 per cent are Rh negative (Rh-). If you are Rh- and your man is Rh+ chances are you are carrying a Rh+ baby. If your baby is Rh+ and his blood mingles with yours (which doesn't usually happen) then you would develop antibodies. You will have frequent blood tests during pregnancy to see if you have any antibodies. If you are clear and having your first baby then there is nothing to be concerned about. Your baby's blood is most likely to mingle with yours at birth (it only happens rarely anyway) and by the time you have developed the antibodies the baby will probably be born. So it wouldn't really affect a first baby.

Within 72 hours of the birth you should have a Rhogam injection that will prevent you developing antibodies which, if untreated, could affect your next baby. This substance is an extremely useful obstetric drug. Before this was invented the Rhesus negative woman could have had great difficulties and sometimes her baby would have needed a complete blood change after birth to clear the antibodies.

Provided you have no antibodies in your blood the pregnancy and birth can take place without any cause for concern. If there are antibodies you would need to deliver in a hospital.

Sex in Pregnancy

See Orgasm.

Sport

Continue with any sport you are good at provided you feel all right about it.

Squash should be avoided as the hard ball could damage the baby. Walking, dancing, jogging (in moderation, and only if you are used to it) and cycling are all suitable, particularly walking and swimming. The latter is especially beneficial, try doing your deep breathing while doing slow breaststroke.

Stitches

See Herbs – herbal bath.
Homoeopathy – calendula tincture.
Perineal Tears or Episiotomy – chapter 7.

Stretch Marks

These are less likely if you stretch during your pregnancy and massage your body regularly with any good vegetable oil.

Thrush

Live yoghurt is very soothing and can help to get rid of thrush (apply locally).

Urinating

In labour: once every hour.
After labour: this can sting if you have a graze or have torn or had an episiotomy. It helps to use a bowl of warm water with some calendula tincture in it.
See Herbal bath.

Varicose Veins

Lots of stretch no. 4 in chapter 2. Do only easy or dictionary squatting – avoid all postures where the legs are compressed. They are caused by weakness in the valves and poor venous return. Stretching will improve the situation.

Water

One of your greatest allies for labour and pregnancy – swim in it, bath in it, shower with it, sponge yourself. When in difficulty – try water.
See Sport.

Recommended Reading

C. Beels, *The Childbirth Book*, Turnstone Press, 1978.

G. S. & T. Brewer, *What Every Pregnant Woman Should Know: The Truth About Diet and Drugs in Pregnancy*, Random House, 1977.

T. Chard & M. Richards, *Benefits and Hazards of the New Obstetrics*, Heinemann Medical Books, 1977.

G. Dick-Read, *Childbirth Without Fear*, Pan, 1969.

Ina May Gaskin, *Spiritual Midwifery*, The Book Publishing Co, 1977 (USA).

Doris Haire, 'The Cultural Warping of Childbirth', in *Environmental Child Health*, Vol. 19, 171–191, June, 1973 (USA).

Sheila Kitzinger, *Birth at Home*, OUP, 1979.

S. Kitzinger, *Experience of Breast Feeding*, Penguin, 1979

S. Kitzinger, *Experience of Childbirth*, Gollancz, 1972; Penguin, 1970.

S. Kitzinger, *Giving Birth*, Sphere, 1979.

S. Kitzinger, *Good Birth Guide*, Fontana, 1979.

S. Kitzinger, *Women as Mothers*, Fontana, 1978.

S. Kitzinger & J. Davis, *The Place of Birth*, OUP, 1978.

La Leche League International, *The Womanly Art of Breastfeeding*, Souvenir Press, 1970; Tandem 1975.

P. Leach, *Baby and Child*, Michael Joseph, 1977; Penguin, 1980.

F. Leboyer, *Birth without Violence*, Fontana, 1977; Alfred A. Knopf, 1978.

F. Leboyer, *Inner Beauty, Inner Light: Yoga for Pregnant Women*, Alfred A. Knopf, 1978.

F. Leboyer, *Loving Hands*, Collins, 1977.

Liedloff, *The Continuum Concept*, Duckworth, 1975; Futura, 1976.

Llewellyn-Jones, D., *Everywoman: A Gynaecological Guide for Life*, Faber, 1978.

G. Lux Flanagan, *The First Nine Months of Life*, Heinemann Medical Books, 1963.

A. Montague, *Touching*, Columbia UP, 1971.

National Childbirth Trust, *Episiotomy – Physical and Emotional Aspects*, 1981.

L. Nilsson, *A Child is Born*, Faber, 1977.

Penny and Andrew Stanway, *Breast is Best*, Pan, 1978.

Useful Addresses

The Active Birth Centre,
   32 Willow Road, Hampstead, NW3.
Association for Improvement in Maternity Services (AIMS),
   Ms Christine Beels, 19 Broomfield Crescent, Leeds 6.
   Elizabeth Cockerell, 10 Stonecliffe View, Farnley, Leeds, LS12 5BE.
Association of Radical Midwives (ARM),
   Lakefield, 8a The Drive, Wimbledon, SW20.
The Birth Centre,
   16 Simpson Street, London, SW11.
British Homoeopathic Association,
   Basildon Court, 27a Devonshire Street, London, W1N 1RT.
La Leche League, Great Britain, (Breastfeeding counsellors),
   Box 3424, London, WC1 6XX.
The Meet-a-Mum Association (MAMA),
   Mary Whitlock, 26a Cumnor Hill, Oxford OX2 9HA.
National Childbirth Trust,
   9 Queensborough Terrace, London, W2 3TB.
National Council for One-Parent Families,
   255 Kentish Town Road, London, NW5 2LX.
The Patients Association,
   11 Dartmouth Street, London, SW1.
   Suffolk House, Banbury Road, Oxford.
Society to Support Home Confinements,
   Margaret Whyte, 17 Laburnam Avenue, Durham.

Index